Introducing Contemporary Psychodynamic Counselling and Psychotherapy

Introducing Contemporary Psychodynamic Counselling and Psychotherapy

The art and science of the unconscious

Alistair Ross

 Open University Press

Open University Press
McGraw-Hill Education
8th Floor, 338 Euston Road
London
England
NW1 3BH

First published 2019

Senior Commissioning Editor: Hannah Kenner
Development Editor: Tom Payne
Editorial Assistant: Karen Harris
Content Product Manager: Ali Davis

A catalogue record of this book is available from the British Library

ISBN-13: 9780335226825
ISBN-10: 0335226825
eISBN: 9780335226832

Library of Congress Cataloging-in-Publication Data
CIP data applied for

Typeset by Transforma Pvt. Ltd., Chennai, India
Printed and bound by CPI Group (UK) Ltd, Croydon, CR0 4YY

Praise for this book

'It is good to see Alistair, a valued student of mine and now an equally valued colleague, taking up the torch for psychodynamic counselling and psychotherapy for a new generation. He has written a book that collates much of the valuable writing to date and at the same time adds new dimensions that should not be overlooked, as fresh ways of understanding psychological development and therapeutic practice influence how even old-stagers like myself think and practise.'

Michael Jacobs, Visiting Professor, University of Leeds and
Bournemouth University, UK

'Ross has emerged over the last decade as one of our leading writers on psychodynamic theory and practice. His engaging style, together with his astute understanding of theory and formidable intellect means his books not only inform a generation of practitioners but contribute to shaping the next. An excellent text that is contemporary and refreshing in equal measure.'

Dr Andrew Reeves, Associate Professor in the Counselling Professions and
Mental Health, University of Chester, UK

'Alistair Ross' book is an excellent comprehensive and lively introduction to psychodynamic ideas and practice. Drawing on his extensive experience as a psychotherapist and trainer, Ross covers a lot of ground without ever compromising on clarity and depth. The book is very up to date with developments within psychoanalysis and it is therefore not only useful to clinicians in training, but also to qualified therapists who could do no better than this book for a contemporary overview of psychodynamic thinking. Highly recommended.'

Prof. Alessandra Lemma, Consultant, Anna Freud National Centre for
Children and Families and Visiting Professor, Psychoanalysis Unit,
University College London, UK

'A welcomed book taking students and practitioners through both the historical nuts and bolts as well as a contemporary analysis of "the art and science of the unconscious". The reader is not only provided with an excellent introduction to contemporary counselling and psychotherapy, but is offered explorations "from chaos, through complexity into a dancing landscape characterised by creativity and connections". Indeed, the author invites us, with his very readable writing style and plentiful helpful vignettes, "to come alive". Could any potential well-adjusted reader's defence mechanisms say "no" to that!'

Prof. Del Loewenthal, Emeritus Professor of Psychotherapy and
Counselling, University of Roehampton, UK

Contents

List of figures and tables

Figures

Tables

Acknowledgements

I have the immense privilege of working with a great staff team, and an ever-changing and growing body of students connected to the Psychodynamic Studies course in the Department for Continuing Education at the University of Oxford.

Many colleagues have read and made comments that have enhanced the text. Special thanks must go to Penny, my administrator, and Nic, who has been, and is, such a good colleague to work with. Thanks also go to Ruth and to Dee who have offered constant support and encouragement. Maureen provided a depth of critical insight that was challenging but so helpful in enabling me to see the wood for the trees in the final stages of writing. Lou and Ali supplied helpful perspectives as working psychodynamic therapists, while Bob introduced me to the wide range of research in a North American context. Tim Bond, Tim Marks, Angie, Ruth, and Sarah have always been great conversation partners for me to try out my ideas. Tom Payne as Development Editor offered insightful comments, especially on Kant. I also want to thank the unnamed clients and supervisees whose composite stories add a vital dimension to the book. While these stories, presented as small vignettes, are fictional, they are based on real therapeutic encounters with clients.

Lastly, thanks must go to my family. To Judy, for allowing me the space, and the many weekends, to write and giving me the opportunity to see something come alive. To my daughter, Hannah, and my son, Toby, who are living their own lives with aliveness and creativity – what more could I ask for or want?

PART 1
Setting the Scene

1

Introduction – the meaning of psychodynamic theory in therapy

This book is about the fascinating and ever-changing world of psychodynamic therapy. As you read through, you will make new discoveries as the text comes alive and speaks directly to you as a trainee or as a working therapist. In doing so, you will be in good company.

The 'father' of psychodynamic therapy is Sigmund Freud. Freud (see the Key Thinkers section for a brief summary) was an avid reader who immersed himself in literature, with a fondness for Shakespeare, and his writing is full of literary references and allusions to life. In his later years, when recuperating from illness or from one of his many operations, he enjoyed reading murder mysteries by Agatha Christie or Dorothy Sayers. Perhaps due to these frequent ailments, we might speculate, Freud was often preoccupied with how we live, how we die, and the struggle to be alive in between. As a psychodynamic therapist myself, I have observed that these Freudian concerns mirror the testimony of my clients and go to the core of every person's existential struggle, summarised in the chimerically simple question, 'What does it mean to be alive?'

In our *external* world, physiologically the answer is obvious: the heart beats, our pulse pulses, blood courses through our veins, and we feel the rhythm of our breathing, with the brain co-ordinating our movements. We are alive. But in another vital place of our existence, our internal world, the answer can be less clear-cut. This is where psychodynamic therapy comes to illuminate and enliven.

What is contemporary psychodynamic therapy?

My first training was as a psychodynamic counsellor. Since Jacobs' early work on psychodynamic counselling (1986, 1988), new ideas have emerged and the context of therapy has changed enormously (Ross 2018). It is important to capture these developments for a new generation of therapists who want to be informed about, and practise, contemporary psychodynamic therapy. Some psychodynamic therapy training programmes use the word 'contemporary' to distinguish them from something that existed previously, but the ideas they incorporate are anything but new. Instead, they rely on the occasional addition of a new ingredient, such as neuroscience, to 'spice things up', all the while harkening to their Freudian psychoanalytical core. That's like adding chilli sauce to spaghetti bolognaise and calling it 'contemporary spag bol' – although, clearly, students have been doing just this for decades. The word 'contemporary' has thus often become a superficial construct when allied to therapy to emphasise the re-packaging of something that *looks* new, but is in essence the same.

Contemporary psychodynamic therapy is, first, a fusion of psychoanalytic ideas drawn from the past. Psychodynamic therapy has Freudian underpinnings and, despite cracks in these foundations, some 'purist' practitioners cling inflexibly to the past, resisting new developments. Although Freud died in 1939, he remains a source of inspiration and there is always something valuable to be found in reading his work and the work of other traditional figures like Jung, Klein, Bion, and Winnicott (see Key Thinkers). Contemporary psychodynamic therapy gives voice to echoes from the past. Second, it is a fusion of newly emerging ideas drawn from intersubjective approaches expressed in *relational* psychoanalysis and *Lacanian* psychoanalysis (see Chapter 12 and Key Thinkers). Third, it is a fusion of ideas that can be valuably applied to psychodynamic working and includes: attachment theory; infant development; neuroscience; new understandings of trauma; and evidence- and practice-based research (Cooper 2008; Green and Latchford 2012). Contemporary psychodynamic therapy, therefore, captures voices from the present. Fourth, and in this respect it is a unique focus, it encourages therapists in training or on-going practice to find their own voice and make their own dynamic fusion. While based on a commonly agreed range of ideas and techniques (see Chapters 13 to 15), the contemporary approach stresses that therapy is yours to construct.

Historically, most therapies have evolved a central orthodoxy, and woe betides you if you departed from the 'truth'. However, the truth of the past and the truth of the present are shaped by a contemporary context where forms of knowledge are more provisional, located in different cultures and contexts, and are constantly changing and this dynamism is appreciated in contemporary psychodynamic therapy. The brave new psychodynamic world is always in a state of flux, moving across old terrain and encountering new landscapes. This is a journey that is creative and chaotic, informed by newly evolving chaos and complexity theories (see Chapter 4), which will enable new forms of contemporary psychodynamic theory and practice to emerge.

What does this mean for contemporary psychodynamic skills?

The skills required for contemporary psychodynamic therapy build on Freud's initial ideas but have expanded as we have learnt more about the working of the mind, consciously and unconsciously. We still rely on transference, counter-transference, and projective processes, but we have evolved more creative and co-constructed ways of being with a client. To understand how this changes our practice with clients, we need to take on board the theoretical developments from the emerging disciplines of infant development and neuroscience. We need to re-examine the changing contexts of gender and sexualities. We need to see the creation of meaning emerging out of socially co-constructed contexts present within the therapy room.

The skills we will develop in Chapters 12 to 15 help us to understand the importance of what is communicated at an assessment stage, consciously and unconsciously, and how nuanced this needs to be. The skills of paying full attention to our clients in our thinking, being, embodiment, eye contact, and tone of voice offer reparative encounters to help clients overcome early emotional (and possibly neurological) deficits in their development. More attention is paid than in the past to building an alliance with the client and fostering an empathic connection. Important new skills include working with intersubjective connections, bearing witness, and attending to the soul. These take account of the whole person, not just their inner world, and help contemporary psychodynamic therapists work with a greater breadth and depth than ever before.

Many of these skills are expressed in the brief clinical vignettes throughout the book that bring theory to life and illustrate the importance of contemporary psychodynamic therapy for a new generation of therapists. Yet there is still much to learn from Freud, so it is with Freud we begin.

Who is this book for?

Whenever Freud wrote, he always had a clear audience in mind. His lectures to his Jewish men's group used accessible language and included many jokes; his lectures to professional medical colleagues introduced new concepts to support the idea of psychoanalysis as a new science. This book has been written with two groups in mind.

The first group is students on psychodynamic or integrative courses who are discovering the wonders of the psychodynamic approach for the first time. This group will be introduced to Freud and key psychodynamic thinkers that evolved his thinking. To make sense of the evolution of psychodynamic thinking, the earlier theoretical chapters provide firm foundations for the latter chapters on practice in the context of psychodynamic theory, while throughout there is a specific focus on the *unconscious* as the unique contribution of a psychodynamic way of understanding. Having established the theoretical foundations of a psychodynamic approach, there will be a focus on using the key skills associated with this approach, drawing on clinical vignettes of psychodynamic therapy in action and offering end-of-chapter reflective questions to help explore the subject further. Relevant key research will be highlighted at the end of each individual chapter, but Chapter 3 is where we examine in depth the contested area of what constitutes research and appropriate (evidence-based) research methods for the field of psychodynamic therapy. In summary, evidence-based research involves a range of methodologies, such as case studies, retrospective studies, mixed-method studies adopting qualitative and quantitative measures, and randomised controlled trials (RCTs). RCTs, which are given primacy in evidence-based research, can be very good for efficacy studies; however, they can be overly exclusive and rigid and encourage research so narrow in scope that its conclusions are less effective with a general range of clients. The research highlighted at the end of most chapters is primarily material available in peer-reviewed and 'credible' research journals, using both qualitative and quantitative methodologies, but the reader will also note practice-based evidence from real cases studies that take us full-circle back to Freud's pioneering research.

The second group is practising psychodynamic or integrative therapists. Many integrative courses teach a psychodynamic component yet understandably such courses often struggle to fit everything in. There is room to learn much more after training as our theoretical understanding comes alive in the clinical setting: it is one thing to talk about transference (see Chapter 13), it is quite another to encounter it with a client and work it through with the aid of good supervision. My material will include new ideas unlikely to have been covered in an original training. Every generation of therapists needs to draw on innovative discoveries about what it is to be with people, working at depth, with the past in the present, in order to forge a new future. This will include new developmental theories and discoveries from the neurosciences. Such new ideas and ways of understanding our clients revitalise therapists and their profession by offering new ways of thinking about our clients.

Coming alive through psychodynamic therapy

Learning from our clients

I believe psychodynamic therapies offer something that is extraordinary. Not only do they 'keep' people alive, but also they 'bring' people alive in a unique way – alive from some unspoken but felt deadness within. This enables clients to feel they are not so utterly alone. Therapists enter into a psychodynamic relational process with their clients where they bring their own experience of tackling life's ultimate questions, doubts, failures, and traumas (Geller et al. 2005). All psychodynamic therapy trainings, counselling psychology, and most integrative trainings require personal therapy to be part of the trainees' experience, a pattern established by Freud (1937). Crucially, trainees face their fears in the supportive context of a therapeutic training and personal therapy. Here is where they encounter a fragile hope, which if nurtured like the sapling of a tree, grows into something deeply rooted, flexible, and strong, giving life and shelter to others. But it is in the engagement with the enigmatic nature of what it means to be 'fully alive' that we are drawn into psychodynamic training and beyond into practice.

Throughout this book, I aim to bring theory to life by referring to clinical vignettes. These are not detailed case studies (commonly found in psychoanalytic papers) but illustrate a key point of theory or technique – they embody the contemporary, non-traditional skills of psychodynamic and integrative therapy. The subtleties of a psychodynamic approach are best learnt relationally through good supervision. Due to the nature of confidentiality, it is ethically unjustifiable to write about specific clinical encounters (unless permission has been given). However, these vignettes come from my experience as a client, therapist, supervisee, and supervisor and are constructed from real words, thoughts, feelings, and emotions. All identifying material has been changed. All names are different. However, some clients want to be spoken about as, consciously, they feel their experience could benefit others, and I suspect unconsciously because they want to remain alive in the therapist's thinking. These glimpses into the space inhabited by therapists and clients serves to reveal the authentic nature of the therapeutic encounter. It also shows how therapists always have something to learn from their patients (Casement 1985, 1990) or from being a patient (Ross 2014, 2016a).

It was a client called May who first taught me the importance of bringing people alive. Her influence has remained with me over the years and informed my subsequent work as a psychodynamic therapist. May's dreams and transference encounters in therapy helped her to make huge progress in her inner world. I introduce May here as it is always important to remind ourselves that clients take centre-stage.

May's story

When I met May, I instinctively thought there was something striking about her. She exuded a bright but fragile air. In her late twenties, she feared that her modelling career was on the slide. Facing competition from younger models, her distinctive 'look' was seen by some in the fashion industry as passé. It emerged over the next few sessions that May did not know who she was. As her external identity was failing, she had begun to look inside and did not like what she saw. At some point, I asked, 'Who are you when you are not a model?', and she replied, 'I am dying from the inside out'. May described how hard she had had to work to build her career as a model after being spotted as a 15-year-old whilst shopping at London's Camden Market. She was signed up by an agency, and then adopted by a well-known fashion house catapulting her career into a whole new stratosphere. Despite a stellar career, May felt her life had been scarred by a series of car-crash relationships. When I explored her early home life she became immensely sad and seemed to shrink into her chair. Sitting in front of me was a six-year-old girl feeling utterly alone, devastated by the divorce of her parents. May blamed herself, wishing she had been a 'better' girl – she thought she could have prevented this disaster from happening.

May learnt the best way of surviving was to do what she was told and bury her feelings. Given that the past shapes the present and, potentially, the future (a key psychodynamic concept explored in Chapter 4), May's childhood survival techniques enabled her to get through to her late twenties but now contributed to her current crisis. The therapy allowed her to discover her buried feelings of rage, repressed into her unconscious, as these were too dangerous to express at the time. The clue to this was in her response to me as her therapist through a process called 'transference' (see Chapters 4, 7, and 13). In brief, this is a process where we are seen 'as if' we are a significant figure from the other person's past. With May, when there was a break in the therapy for a holiday or some other event, the session on return was volcanic in intensity and emotion. She would rage at me as I became seen as if I were another abandoning figure: '[You're] just like my parents, you're no better. And I'm even paying you for this crap'. The repressed feelings May had previously had about her parents were being 'transferred' onto me, thus giving me a clue as to how abandoned and angry May felt as a child, a pattern that she was re-working in her adult relationships.

In discovering she could express her rage and not be abandoned, May began to take risks in relationships. She began to bring dreams to our session where together we uncovered what these could mean about her inner world. May had woken up from a long sleep to discover who she was, both on the inside and the outside.

We finished our work and May went onto university, her long-standing dream. Unexpectedly, I received a letter after her graduation where she told me that she had met someone, now her partner, a relationship she experienced as affirming and challenging. I have not heard from her since, yet from time to time I wonder how she is getting on. Fifteen years later, I happened upon May on the cover of a magazine. The fragile air she once possessed was replaced by a self-assured confidence, and most importantly she looked content.

Learning from my experience

Several years ago, in 2014, I had a very serious, potentially life-threatening fall down a mountain. This had a number of vital consequences. I decided I only wanted to write about what I was passionate about, which makes this book a very personal introduction to psychodynamic therapy. As I wrote, this event and my associated feelings kept emerging in the text. My voice and its passions will clearly be heard. I also use illustrations from my own life and work, and often include analogies related to walking in the hills and mountains of Scotland and Wales. Underlying this is a desire that you, the reader, develop your own therapeutic voice, whether psychodynamic, integrative, as a trainee, or as a working therapist.

The following chapters will help you. But, like all the best stories, the best place to begin is at the beginning.

Reflective questions

What struck you about May's story?

Who, or what, informs your current thinking and work as a current or aspiring therapist?

What key areas do you want to develop in?

What is the one thought you will take away from reading this introductory chapter?

Looking at research

(Surveying the field as a whole, including psychodynamic approaches)

Cooper, M. (2008) *Essential Research Findings in Counselling and Psychotherapy*. London: SAGE.

Fonagy, P., Cotterell, D., Phillips, J., Bevington, D., Glaser, D. and Allison, E. (2016) *What Works for Whom? A Critical Review of Treatments for Children and Adolescents*, 2nd edn. New York: Guilford Press.

Roth, A. and Fonagy, P. (2005) *What Works for Whom? A Critical Review of Psychotherapy Research*, 2nd edn. New York: Guilford Press.

Timulak, L. (2009) *Research in Psychotherapy and Counselling*. London: SAGE.

2

Understanding the past – how did we get here?

This chapter tells the story of how Freud, his ideas, and his clinical practices evolved into psychoanalysis and initiated the new disciplines of psychotherapy, counselling, and psychodynamic counselling. Psychodynamic ideas and techniques are so influential, and self-evidently true, they are incorporated into integrative forms of counselling, psychotherapy, counselling psychology, and other cognitive therapeutic approaches. This chapter examines how these strands evolved, converged, and diverged as part of the therapeutic landscape we inhabit today.

What do we owe Freud?

We all have a birthday, a birthplace, and a birth certificate. We know we exist and have an official document to prove it – but it doesn't answer such existential questions as, 'Who am I?', 'Where did I come from (often meaning *who* did I come from)?', and 'How does my past determine my present?' These same questions can be asked of psychotherapy. Freud really is the 'father' of psychotherapy and all therapies can trace their origins to Freud, either as part of the psychodynamic family or in reaction against Freud and his ideas, like a newly constituted step-family. Sayers (1991) points out there are many mothers in psychoanalysis as well, figures who have continued to give birth to new ideas and techniques. Yet, psychoanalysis began with Freud who polarised and energised people to think in radically new ways. The markers of his DNA can be found in all dynamic-based therapies, so it is important to start with a brief history to discover more about our kith and kin. We can do this through examining the following terms: psychodynamic; psychoanalysis; psychotherapy; counselling; and psychodynamic counselling.

Psychodynamic

The word 'psychodynamic', like conjoined twins, combines two meanings in one form.

The first part, 'psycho', comes from the Greek word *psykhe*. It referred originally to Psykhe, the goddess of the soul in Greek mythology, who is purified by searching for passion and overcoming misfortunes to be prepared for true happiness and love. C.S. Lewis's re-telling of the story of Psykhe and Cupid (1956) delves into the obsessive and scarring experiences of what it is to love, encounter injustice, passion, guilt, shame, and aloneness – the stuff of psychoanalysis. Freud used the word 'psyche' in general to refer to the soul in a secular sense, focusing on the human spirit or mind and in particular the conscious and unconscious processes that fulfil or frustrate how we become a person in relation to ourselves and to others. Freud called the analysis of the psyche 'psychoanalysis'.

The second part, 'dynamic', refers to constant activity and the flux of movement and time in the psyche. Imagine sitting on the sea-shore, watching the ebb and flow of white-plumed waves as they crash over rocks, spraying water into ever-changing shapes, infusing a salt-tang to the air. Likewise, the psyche is in constant flux expressed by an internal world that is both conscious and unconscious; our external world, the place we inhabit; the relationships that hold these two worlds together – past and present; and our mercurial emotions and how we engage with them through our loves, losses, hopes, fears, creativities, and fantasies.

When you fuse these two ideas together to form 'psychodynamic', it conveys the meaning of the interrelationship and activity between different aspects of the individual's psyche – mind, spirit, emotion, soul – in a way that is irrepressibly *alive*. A key figure initiating this new way of understanding the self was Freud.

Psychoanalysis

Freud's life-story is fascinating and well worth exploring in detail, not least because it gives us clues to the origins of psychoanalysis (Ross 2016b). Freud tells us he discovered psychoanalysis through a dream after the death of his father. Like IKEA furniture, psychoanalysis arrived in pieces with vaguely helpful instructions, and possibly one or two components missing. It took several attempts to assemble, but what Freud discovered gripped him and he wrote about it and lived it out for the rest of his life. Freud's single Viennese flat-pack furniture became a fully assembled Huf Haus, a dream home in the Bauhaus tradition. Building on some pre-existing ideas but uniquely adapted and assembled by Freud along with genuinely new components, psychoanalysis altered the trajectory of thinking and culture in the twentieth and twenty-first centuries and new orbits are still being explored today.

Freud's psychoanalysis, as well as being a theory of the mind and a developmental process, was a set of therapeutic techniques aimed at relieving the suffering patient. These consisted of seeing a patient (analysand) six times a week (exceptions being made for Sunday, public holidays, and a summer break) over a period of several years. Freud made exceptions for people he had treated before whose treatment was satisfactorily advanced: he saw them three times a week (Freud 1913). Very occasionally, Freud saw people for a single consultation with great effect (Ross 2016e). We see one such instance in the experience of the composer Gustav Mahler who travelled to meet Freud, despite Freud being on holiday in the Netherlands. They only met once but this encounter, as they walked around Leiden for several hours, brought Mahler happiness in the last year of his life. Freud also saw patients, often people wanting to become analysts from overseas, who could only be in Vienna for several months. Freud's patients would attend his consulting room at Bergasse 19 and were invited to lie on a couch, with Freud sitting on a chair at one end, out of the line of sight. While he might have been smoking a cigar, he would not have been taking notes, as portrayed in cartoons. They would tell Freud their symptoms and were encouraged to 'free associate': to say the first things that came to mind without censorship.

Freud encouraged his patients to imagine they were looking out the carriage window when on a train journey and describe the changing scenery (1913). Resistance to this, experienced as forgetting or the mind going blank, gives the analyst insight into unconscious processes at work. The unconscious is also explored through describing one's dreams and the analyst offering interpretations of the complex, disguised, and condensed elements in the dream. Thus the patient gains insight into their inner world – their unconscious motivations are freed from aspects of the past, and they are enabled to make better choices for the future. As psychoanalysis developed, four or five sessions weekly became the norm deemed necessary to reach the most hidden aspects of a person. Psychoanalytic societies and training institutes emerged across Europe, Britain, and the USA, all belonging to the International Psychoanalytical Association (Loewenberg and Thompson 2011). Over time, psychoanalysis was adapted to become psychoanalytic psychotherapy and psychodynamic counselling, to which we now turn.

Psychotherapy

Therapy or psychological therapies are the current, inclusive terms used to refer to a wide range of psychological treatments including psychoanalysis, psychotherapy, counselling, and cognitive approaches. In the beginning, long before psychoanalysis was even a gleam in Freud's eye, there were people who offered support, healing, insight, care, dream interpretation, knowledge, or wisdom to those who needed help (Ellenberger 1970). They often had a title as recognition of their role in the tribe, community, or religion such as 'elder', 'priest', or 'wise woman'. So psychotherapy, broadly understood, existed before Freud, but psychoanalysis changed everything. Freud's radical shift of focus was to examine the unconscious drives of the internal world rather than external circumstances. Freud described his earliest work as 'hypnotic psychotherapy' but, as his ideas and techniques evolved into psychoanalysis, he clearly distinguished psychotherapy from psychoanalysis (1905b). He recognised physicians dealt with patients through a broadly defined helping relationship termed 'psychotherapy', but for Freud this was superseded by psychoanalysis. This alone could get to the depths people required.

With the First World War and the advent of what was termed 'shell shock', Freud's ideas of unconscious processes and the body's capacity to express emotional trauma (Brunner 1991) were applied in non-clinical settings by British psychiatrists such as Bernard Hart and W.H.R. Rivers (Kuhn 2016). Psychiatrists, who were on the front-line of treatment in military hospitals, continued to use psychotherapy but incorporated a briefer form of psychoanalysis that was not solely focused on the unconscious life, principally driven by sexuality (Hart 1916). The term 'new psychology' came into popular use to describe these evolving therapeutic interests including the founding of the Tavistock Clinic in London in 1920, offering therapy less frequently and over a shorter period than psychoanalysis to people on limited incomes. Psychotherapy developed through diverse strands of practice such as these rather than becoming a separate and defined profession. It was often a speciality developed after a person had been in analysis in order to utilise this experience alongside their professional role (for example, doctor, psychiatrist, social worker, probation officer, psychologist, clergy, and the like). Tavistock continued to grow, exerting a considerable influence on psychoanalysis outside the consulting room (Dicks 1970). Another development was the promotion of Jungian ideas through the C.G. Jung Club, which formed in London in 1923; the Guild of Pastoral Psycho-Therapy (now the Guild of

Pastoral Psychology) in 1936; and the Society of Analytic Psychology (SAP) in 1946, which offered a low-cost clinic and a training programme for Jungian analysts and psychotherapists. Psychoanalytic and Jungian societies and their training institutes carefully guarded their analytic terrain and exclusive membership (Scarlett 1991).

The aftermath of the Second World War also offered new opportunities for psychotherapy (Jones 2004). A desire to build for a new and better future led to the creation of a National Health Service (NHS) in Britain in 1948. In 1950, two clusters of psychotherapists began clinical case discussion groups in Oxford and London and these influenced the formation of the Association of Psychotherapists in 1951. All training members of this new association were required to have Freudian or Jungian analysis (three times a week), plus the opportunity to acquire clinical experience. Becoming the British Association of Psychotherapists in 1972, this gave psychotherapy a place to belong, albeit of predominately psychoanalytic bent. Psychotherapy subsequently branched out into many other forms including child guidance, child psychotherapy, educational psychology, marriage guidance, social work, organisational consultancy, and group analysis (Jones 2004).

Psychotherapy has come a long way from its psychodynamic origins, now incorporating a very diverse range of therapies, linked by a desire to be professional, ethical, and accountable, whilst sharing a vision for the psychological health and well-being of individuals and society.

Counselling

Religious traditions have long histories of pastoral counsel (Oden 1987) where an important role for a spiritual leader is to help people come to terms with life-events and losses, discovering comfort and meaning. During the First World War, chaplains serving in the trenches were confronted by many harsh realities and saw shell shock first hand. On returning to their church contexts and with the help of 'new psychology', they combined faith with psychological and psychoanalytic insights (Pym 1922). Later developments in pastoral counselling came through the work of psychiatrist Frank Lake, who established the Clinical Theology Association in 1958 and published a seminal text *Clinical Theology* (1966). Lake combined Christian theology with ideas from Guntrip (his teacher) and Klein (see Key Thinkers), delivered through experiential groups. His work was the most important influence on pastoral counselling throughout the 1960s and 1970s, leading many clergy and lay-people to seek further training as counsellors and psychotherapists (Ross 1993).

Another major influence in the development of counselling in Britain came from the USA in the person of Carl Rogers, taken up by Mearns and Thorne (Thorne 2007). Rogers' work in the 1930s with children who had behavioural problems and their parent(s) led him to move away from a diagnostic, expert stance that he felt removed him from the emotional needs appearing in front of him. He began to listen and stopped interpreting. Rogers, who later developed his ideas in *Client-centered Therapy* (1951) and *On Becoming a Person* (1961), reacted against the disempowerment of viewing the patient as someone who needed to be told what was going on in their unconscious by the analyst. This came at a time when, in the USA at least, psychoanalysis was the dominant force in psychiatry and psychotherapy. Rogers' research, theory, and clinical practice during the 1940s and 1950s put the patient, re-named the 'client', at the centre and he argued anyone, given the core conditions of empathy, congruence, and unconditional positive regard, could thrive and grow, becoming resourceful enough to overcome their own problems. These resources come from within the client, encouraged by the counsellor rather than from any expert insight or interpretation. (This approach to counselling proved very popular and expanded into marriage guidance, social work, and work in schools.) A significant step in the development of counselling was the establishing of training courses at Keele and Reading universities in 1964 facilitated by visiting Fulbright scholars from the USA, steeped in Rogers' ideas.

Where counselling differed immensely from psychoanalysis and psychotherapy was on the understanding of the social context and the external world of the client. The vision of many coming into the counselling profession was of a transforming movement that could give power and authority back to ordinary people rather than remaining in the hands of experts (Aldridge 2014). By the early 1970s, counselling flourished with the evolution of university counselling services, counselling provision in the voluntary sector, and a fascination with new experiential, humanistic, personal growth-focused therapies coming from West Coast America (Clare and Thompson 1981). New professional groupings and associations emerged that led to the establishment of the British Association for Counselling in 1977 (now BACP, with the addition of psychotherapy in 2000). Within these exciting new developments, a unique hybrid emerged in the form of psychodynamic counselling that spanned the best of these counselling and psychotherapy traditions.

Psychodynamic counselling

This was a creative development that combined psychoanalytic and psychotherapeutic ideas and techniques, applied within a counselling framework (Ross 2018). This framework balanced the inner and outer worlds of the client, rather than solely concentrating on the psyche. Psychodynamic counselling focused as much on personal growth as it did on dealing with personal psychopathology. It normally took place once a week, as a face-to-face encounter, with the person receiving the counselling referred to as a 'client' (rather than a patient).

There were several distinctive strands that formed the basis of psychodynamic counselling.

- The first strand was the Tavistock Clinic establishing a Young People's Counselling Service in the late 1950s, based on psychodynamic principles.
- The second strand was Balint's brief psychotherapy workshops working alongside Malan, whose research at the Tavistock established a rationale for briefer forms of psychodynamic therapy (Malan 1979) that influenced the development of short-term dynamic therapy (Coren 2010).
- The third strand was the development of student counselling in 1972, and the first training course being based on psychodynamic ideas led by Noonan at the extramural department of London University, now Birkbeck (Noonan 2003).
- The fourth strand came from pastoral counselling. The Westminster Pastoral Foundation (WPF), established in 1969, offered psychodynamic counselling and training. Lee's *Principles of Pastoral Counselling* (1968) and Jacobs' *Still Small Voice* (1982) were popular texts that adopted a psychodynamic approach.

In the 1980s, Jacobs wrote two influential books, *The Presenting Past* and *Psychodynamic Counselling in Action* (1986, 1988), which gave a clearer identity to psychodynamic counselling. Jacobs was particularly influential in my development when I began integrating Freud with a Christian faith perspective through the object relations ideas of Guntrip and Winnicott. (Later, this led to my doctoral research on what I called 'sacred psychoanalysis' [Ross 2010].) Psychodynamic counselling made psychoanalytic ideas much more available and accessible throughout the UK. Psychodynamic counselling training courses emerged in London, Oxford, Cambridge, Leicester, Birmingham, and Edinburgh alongside a range of courses across southern England linked with the WPF.

Current developments

The worlds of counselling and psychotherapy are in continual and dynamic flux. Since the 1980s, professional bodies have emerged to promote the counselling and psychotherapy profession including the United Kingdom Council for Psychotherapy (UKCP), the British Psychoanalytic Council (BPC), and the British Association for Counselling and Psychotherapy (BACP) whose vision and values are captured in their *Ethical Framework for the Counselling Professions* (Bond 2018). Alongside national bodies, devolved psychotherapy organisations have emerged such as Counselling and Psychotherapy in Scotland (COSCA) and specific trainings including Relate's College of Sexual and Relationship Therapists (COSRT).

Alongside these professional bodies, counselling and psychotherapy have seen pivotal theoretical developments, such as the combining of different theoretical approaches under the umbrella term, 'integration'. An integrative therapist might use a psychodynamic idea like the past influencing the present, with a person-centred idea of staying in the present moment of the therapeutic encounter; and they might offer a cognitive re-framing of a problem whilst focusing on a solution. Such integration combines multiple therapeutic approaches in one adaptive personal model, tailoring these depending on the needs of the client. There are many forms of integrative approaches that have been around for a long time, but from the 1990s onwards there was a significant growth in the number of therapists being trained in these methods (Hollanders 2007). A parallel development was the emergence of a range of cognitive-based therapies, the most common being cognitive behavioural therapy (CBT). This takes a very different stance from a psychodynamic approach. A client experiencing anxiety or depression wants relief from the debilitating impact of these conditions now, not after months or years of therapy. CBT posits that change is not dependent on the resolution of long-standing difficulties but can begin immediately. If the problem is expressed in negative cognitions and behaviours, these can be addressed. As CBT developed, it garnered a strong research base measuring outcomes and effectiveness quantitatively (Roth and Fonagy 2005). Adopting a manualised form of training alongside specific cognitive interventions increased the ease with which CBT practitioners could be trained.

This fitted with the *zeitgeist* of evidence-based medicine, something we see a resurgence of today (see Chapter 3). When the economic benefit of getting people back into the workforce more quickly was estimated, the government funded a programme to make cognitive interventions (drawn from CBT) accessible to as many people as possible through the NHS (Improving Access to Psychological Therapies, IAPT). The unspoken cost was the impact of a reductive, non-nuanced vision of people's psychological needs. This has changed the therapeutic landscape beyond recognition. How can we understand this complex therapeutic scene? An answer can be found in another new development: the emergence of complexity theory.

Summary

Freud's psychoanalysis spawned many imitators and rivals. Whether they are grouped under psychotherapy, counselling, counselling psychology, integrative counselling, CBT, or psychodynamic counselling, each approach has its individual history and integrity in its quest to meet the needs of people in psychological and psychic pain. It is too easy to split into tribal battles that have beset the history of psychological therapies throughout the world. Future co-operation requires knowing where we have come from, what has divided us in the past, and acknowledging what can unite us for the future to improve the outcomes of our clients.

Reflective questions

How does knowing the roots of your therapeutic approach help you understand counselling and psychotherapy today?

What might have been the missed opportunities to work together?

Where do you fit within this therapeutic landscape?

Looking at research

An important text is Norcross's *Psychotherapy Relationships that Work: Evidence-based Responsiveness* (2011), although a limitation is the lack of clinical case studies. He takes a trans-theoretical approach, which can be balanced with an online resource from the BPC. Available at:

https://www.bpc.org.uk/sites/psychoanalytic-council.org/files/FINAL%20Overview_Evidence_Base_Briefing.pdf [accessed 13 November 2018].

3

Understanding the present –
the role of research

Research changes lives and the way we view the world. It shapes opinions, influences policies and practices, creates new ideas, and enhances clinical techniques. This chapter explores the nature of, and challenges associated with, the research evidence that supports a psychodynamic way of doing therapy. Without evidence, we become mere custodians passing down beliefs, rituals, and practices from the past, rather than ensuring the best possible outcomes for our clients. (Using a landscape model [see Chapter 4], this marks a shift from a fixed landscape to a dancing landscape, where new and old possibilities emerge and re-emerge.) All therapy should be able to withstand rigorous scrutiny from different philosophical, medical, or clinical perspectives, as well as taking into account evidence generated in different ways.

Obstacles to research

Dan and Karin's story

I met Dan and Karin on holiday in Umbria. Over a few bottles of wine, I learnt they were both teachers in second marriages and they learnt I was an academic and psycho-dynamic therapist. Karin blurted out, 'So you see people lying on a couch'. I explained not but she went on to say her first husband had spent a fortune on four years of four-time-weekly analysis.

'It didn't help, he still slept with other women, and then he left so it was worth every penny. I want to know, does it work?'

I replied that it does work but maybe not in the way they expected, as at least he had left leaving her free to make a new relationship. Both Dan and Karin loved this idea.

Karin's question 'does it work?' seems simple enough but it takes us into complex and contested territory. Roth and Fonagy (2005), Cooper (2008), Norcross (2011), Wampold and Imel (2015), and Cozolino (2016) attempt to answer this vital question. They summarise an amazing breadth of research evidence and provide a good foundation to build on. In addition, there are many high-quality counselling and psychotherapy research journals where articles are peer-reviewed. The problem is that purchasing individual articles can be costly, although some articles can be obtained through a free or reduced price open access policy. *ResearchGate*, for example, brings researchers together and offers an online community where you can request texts from the author, follow the research of others, receive alerts, and ask questions. This is invaluable, as there is little point in doing research if it then languishes in some dank, forgotten repository. Research needs to become known, used, adapted, disagreed with, updated, replaced, replicated, all in the cause of understanding, in more breadth and depth, what happens in the therapeutic process for the benefit of therapist and client (Reeves 2014).

So what do we do with this research? Research provides an evidence base that is used to shape the provision of therapy in publicly- or insurance-funded healthcare systems. These adopt a utilitarian approach about what offers the best for the many. However, the calculations used to determine this and the principles behind this approach are open to debate. In the UK, the National Institute for Health and Care Excellence (NICE) offers guidelines that determine clinical priorities and the commissioning of services. In the USA, the National Institutes of Health (NIH) fund research that guides policy development and provision with the aim of turning discovery into health. These and other bodies reveal a bias towards research that utilises randomised control trials (RCTs) and quantitative (statistical) analysis (Arean and Kraemer 2013). This bias, enforced by the selective allocation of funds, can lead to the neglect of practice-based evidence involving case-study research (McLeod 2010) or practitioner research (Bondi and Fewell 2016) as well as a discounting of psychotherapy or counselling as effective interventions. Research that demonstrates the effectiveness of counselling and psychotherapy is vitally important as long as effectiveness is interpreted in the widest sense of a person's well-being (Shedler 2010, 2017; Gazzillo et al. 2017) rather than being reduced to a score on an evaluation form. Based on current qualitative and quantitative research, it is possible to make a 'good-enough' case to support key aspects found in all therapies and specific aspects found in dynamic therapies, an important point made by the former National Professional Adviser for Improving Access to Psychological Therapies (2008–2013), Jeremy Clarke (2018). Historically, NICE acknowledged the importance of client perspectives in the development of evidence-based practice, but these have often been neglected. A recovery of this could lead to a more nuanced evidence base and allow greater recognition of qualitative rather than just quantitative methodologies.

The context of research

There are four issues we need to bear in mind in understanding the research landscape today. The first is that historically psychoanalysis and subsequent dynamic therapies have been resistant to getting involved in research. Despite this, it has still taken place, as Robert Gordon illustrates:

> Empirical research in psychoanalysis began early on. Otto Fenichel in 1930 studied the results of 721 patients in psychoanalysis at the Berlin Institute. He found that psychoanalysis was very effective for the neurotic patients, but not so effective for the psychotic patients. Psychoanalytic researchers continued publishing empirical effectiveness

and process studies with refinements in theory and treatment over the years. Although this research has been largely ignored by academic psychologists.

(2010: 22)

Second, compared with the sample sizes in large-scale quantitative research found in psychology and cognitive-based research, the numbers involved for qualitative research in counselling or psychotherapy are often small (McLeod 2016). The aim of qualitative research, however, is not to produce a representative sample across a whole population. Qualitative research focuses on an in-depth experience of a small number of people, clients, or therapist (Ross and Green 2011). Informed debate needs to balance breadth with depth.

The third issue is that, in order to get a sufficiently homogeneous group to research, every study has exclusion criteria. For example, in researching eating disorders, people who have a pre-existing history of sexual abuse or mental health difficulties would be excluded so that the results can say, in essence, 'This treatment is statistically effective with this group with this disorder at this time'. The reality is that the clients we see are more complex than the eating disorder they present with, so all research needs to be contextualised, interpreted, and applied bearing in mind that, where there are strict exclusion criteria, we may not see the promised results with all clients.

Fourth, the nature of the unconscious makes it difficult, but not impossible, to research (Gordon 2001). Gordon later writes:

Psychodynamic researchers wanted to study complex syndromes that involved affects, memories, cognitions, behaviors, preconscious fantasies, temperament, attachment and object internalizations and defenses in a dynamic interaction. They were interested in studying polysymptomatic patients with underlying personality disorders that are common to actual practice, as well as assessing increasing mental capacities such as ego resiliency.

(2010: 22)

Sometimes our clients are too complex. Sometimes there are too many variables to produce 'clean' empirical research. Yet it is a challenge we must take up for the future good of clients.

Learning the language

Research is a new language that contemporary psychodynamic therapists need to learn in order to best help clients. An on-going debate in psychodynamic therapies is whether it is a form of treatment expressed in symptom reduction or a way of making meaning about the complex and chaotic internal world that threatens to overwhelm. Even if we favour the latter, we can still be aware of how research can support this task. For example, in Chapters 9 and 10, we will survey new developments in infant development based on observations and research. This has direct implications for practice. We saw how finely tuned people are. The very stance we take, the way we sit, the manner in which we look at our clients – holding their gaze without judgement – the tone and inflection of our voice, allied to a consistency and reliability of weekly or twice-weekly encounters, all communicate at a profound, pre-verbal level. This can be deeply reparative, as I have found personally in several different forms of dynamic therapy. We can give someone whose inner object world is barren or depleted and who can get caught up in their basic fault a new experience of the bonds of love. Both qualitative and quantitative research suggests that all therapies, irrespective of modality, and their associated skill sets are more effective if they can develop and maintain the following six aspects.

The six aspects of effective therapy

Client motivation and involvement

I once worked for an Employee Assistance Programme (EAP) and was 'sent' clients who had been 'told' by their manager to attend, with some unspoken implications if they did not. The first session was always about getting the person to view therapy as something for them rather than some form of punishment. I was attempting to get them motivated and involved. I did not enjoy this work and left after six months.

Involving the client has been shown to be one of the most significant predictors of a positive outcome from therapy (Cooper 2008) – therapy is something clients do, not something that is done to them. This may take the form of an agreed focus or goal as found in one aspect of the therapeutic alliance. Dynamic Interpersonal Therapy (DIT) (Lemma et al. 2011) takes this further by adding one key interpersonal relationship and my experience as a DIT therapist saw clients make significant progress. Reduced scores in a widely used research tool, Clinical Outcomes and Routine Evaluation Outcome Measure (CORE-OM), confirmed my subjective experience. CORE-OM is a client self-report questionnaire completed before and after therapy. The client is asked 34 questions about how they have felt over the last week, using a five-point scale ranging from 'not at all' to 'most or all of the time'. The questionnaire covers subjective well-being, problems/symptoms, life functioning, and risk/harm. CORE-OM has developed different versions including shorter forms and one for young people. It is a very useful tool illustrating how research can routinely be done with clients in a way that provides evidence of improvement, supported by over 200 research papers, articles, chapters, audits, and books (http://www.coreims.co.uk/Downloads_References.html [accessed 19 October 2018]).

A therapeutic, helping, or working alliance

If you have ever been in therapy, stop and ask yourself this question: 'Do I think or feel my therapist liked me?' I appreciate some may not feel this is a fair question but it points directly to the importance of the quality of the relationship and how this was communicated to you, the client. Freud understood this and, in the last years of his life, he re-examined techniques covering transference, repression, resistance, and the quality of the relationship between clients and therapists (1938). He concluded it was the ability to encounter positive and negative transference in a collaborative way that allows a re-working of the past and enables the person to find a new freedom in the present. Bordin (1979) identified that no matter what unconscious processes and techniques were at work, there needed to be a conscious, working relationship or bond between client and therapist. He identified three parts of an effective therapeutic relationship: therapist and client agreement on goals; therapist and client consensus on the process and tasks of therapy; and a mutual bond based on trust and acceptance. Horvath and Greenberg's (1989) 'Working Alliance Inventory' has become a widely used measure revealing the quality of the alliance as the best predictor of clients valuing and completing therapy (Roth and Fonagy 2005), and we see a similar idea expressed by Cooper:

> Measures of the alliance in the early stages of therapy . . . (the third to fifth sessions) are especially strong predictors of positive therapeutic outcomes . . . this suggests that therapy should be particularly mindful of establishing a strong collaborative relationship in the first few sessions . . . the highest priority in the early phases of therapy.
>
> (2008: 104)

An appropriate match between client and therapist (based on therapeutic modality and client issue/problem/condition)

While this would make logical sense, Roth and Fonagy reveal there is limited research in this area:

> The research related to dynamic therapies includes studies that] have examined the impact on outcome of patients' 'quality of object relations' and psychological minded-ness . . . Patients with higher levels of motivation . . . and a more stable and coherent sense of self responded better to dynamic explorations of their difficulties . . . patients who describe their problems more in terms of interpersonal difficulties than symptoms tend to have better outcomes in psychodynamic psychotherapy.
>
> (2005: 470)

Fonagy (2010), in interpreting Watzke and colleagues' (2010) research, proposes that in order for psychodynamic therapy to be most effective, there needs to be an appropriate selection of clients. Used generally across a whole population, cognitive behavioural therapies appeared more effective, but for people wanting and able to work with a dynamic approach, there was a greater impact. In research on clients with borderline issues, both cognitive and dynamic therapies were effective, particularly mentalisation; however, improvements were maintained over a longer period of time using dynamic therapies (Bateman and Fonagy 2008, 2009). This suggests that matching specific clients or client groups to specific psychodynamic therapies would benefit clients.

A relationship in which the client feels the therapist is interested in, empathic towards, or curious about them

This is an extension of the bonds Bordin discusses in the working alliance and, while empathy is traditionally associated with Rogers' person-centred therapy, a consequence of our growing knowledge from developmental research is the vital importance of an *empathic attunement*. Applied psychodynamically, empathic therapists help clients by putting their experience into words while noting their emotional responses, as therapist and client. This enables clients to experience what these words mean by examining their thoughts and feelings. Dynamic therapists also pay great attention to what is not said, existing at the periphery of awareness, waiting to be given voice.

Zoe's story

Using research from my private practice, I utilise a working alliance measure the client completes every session. Zoe, a 19-year-old, came with diagnoses of borderline personality disorder, bulimia, self-harm behaviours, and suicidal ideation. Zoe was on various prescribed drugs and I obtained her permission to contact her GP if required. Each week, she completed a self-report PHQ-9 form rating depression (https://www.nhs.uk/Tools/Documents/Mood%20self-assessment.htm) and a simplified working alliance form. If the client scores low in certain areas, this raises a 'red flag' that something is need of attention. When Zoe answered the question, 'My therapist seemed pleased to see me', with a middle score on a Likert rating scale, this indicated a red flag issue, so I raised this with her (in session five). She laughed, saying, 'I came to see you because you had a reputation for being professional and not very friendly. I saw a previous counsellor who was all very "flowery" and said I could say anything I wanted but when I did, like I was suicidal, she went all panicky trying to reassure me. I thought I can't tell her the real truth. Here I tell you the truth, you don't panic, you treat me the same, you don't get shocked, which makes me feel safe – but I don't want to be your friend'.

Zoe gave me permission to talk or write about her 'unfriendly therapist'. Zoe felt that I was interested in and curious about her, enabling her to be curious about aspects of her life in the past, and the things she said and did in the present.

The spotting of and dealing with ruptures in the therapeutic relationship

A rupture is a tension or a tear in the therapeutic alliance. This can range from differing levels of understanding and engagement that is experienced as psychological discomfort, to a fundamental relational mismatch. It could become a total breakdown if the client feels excessively misunderstood, imposed upon, criticised, or that their therapist doesn't like them. Transferential processes at work, as illustrated in May's story in Chapter 1, further complicate this, so it is essential that a good working alliance is in place to weather these storms. Yet sometimes it is just not possible. It is also important that, if a therapist has made a mistake, they acknowledge this. While linked to the therapeutic alliance (Safran 2012), there is evidence that identifying a rupture and addressing it is essential for on-going therapeutic engagement (Safran and Muran 2000; Safran et al. 2011), or in dealing with an impasse or setback (Leiper and Kent 2001).

My story; Wendy's story

I once called a client, Wendy, the wrong name, not just once but twice in the same session. Without any awareness on my part, it was the same name as her best friend towards whom she felt rivalrous. Supervision enabled me to identify what unconscious processes were going on but the relationship with the client needed to be repaired the

> very next session. I apologised and did not try to explain it away by talking about the unconscious. Instead, we worked with what feelings Wendy had, both about her and about me, and what enactment had taken place. Her words were not flattering but we worked together for a further eight sessions. My mistake unearthed a degree of ambivalence in Wendy who both wanted, and didn't want, therapy. In a final session, Wendy declared, 'I had to decide between therapy and shoes. Shoes won'.

Allowing sufficient time

Research suggests that therapy takes time to show effectiveness, a factor that is rarely captured in RCT-focused research. Shedler (2017) sums up the situation following the publication of new trauma guidelines in the USA.

> Psychotherapy takes time. Psychotherapy follows a 'dose–response' curve. It takes more than 20 sessions, or about 6 months of weekly therapy, before 50% of patients show clinically-meaningful improvement. It takes more than 40 sessions before 75% of patients show meaningful improvement. These findings, based on scientific study of more than 10,000 therapy cases, dovetail with what therapists report about successful treatments and what patients report about their own therapy experiences.

Some RCTs that reveal long-term effectiveness are on mentalisation, where the effectiveness of dynamic therapies is maintained over a longer period of time compared with cognitive interventions (Bateman and Fonagy 2008, 2009), and dynamic therapies have a positive impact on families and partners of clients with a borderline diagnosis (Bateman and Fonagy 2018). Similar results about long-term effectiveness were found in a seven-year follow-up study of clients with personality disorder using group psychotherapy (Fjeldstad et al. 2016).

What research supports psychodynamic clinical techniques?

Freud's observations of his patients were the original form case-study research and demonstrate the value of practice-based evidence. In the past, psychoanalysis has been resistant to engage in research – however, this is changing. Fonagy and Target (1996) conducted a retrospective review of the treatment of 763 children given therapy at the Anna Freud Centre. Three-quarters showed improvement (statistically and clinically) when treatment lasted more than six months and, while psychotherapy and psychoanalysis were both effective, psychoanalysis was even more effective with children presenting with the most severe problems. In 2000, Sandell (and team) published results from the Stockholm Outcome of Psychoanalysis and Psychotherapy Project. This naturalistic outcome study (not an RCT) used interviews, questionnaires, and statistical data to determine the impact of psychoanalysis, or long-term psychotherapy, on 400 clients over a three-year period. Using self-rating measures, both were effective for symptom relief and morale, but both were equally weak for social relations. The explanation of the differences in results between clients in psychoanalysis and psychotherapy related to therapist factors. Psychodynamic therapists adopting a psychoanalytic approach, without the benefit of being grounded in psychoanalytic training, were less effective, although still helpful for the client. Is the solution to get everyone to train as a psychoanalyst, then? That is not an affordable or practical option. Rather, therapists ought not to 'recycle' psychoanalytic ideas but rather adopt newly emerging interdisciplinary ideas (e.g. neuroscience) and have confidence in contemporary psychodynamic therapy (Sandell 2012).

Another key study came from Shedler (2010), who evaluated eight meta-analyses demonstrating the efficacy of dynamic therapies. These included RCTs and control studies (e.g. cognitive behavioural therapy, CBT) covering depression, anxiety, eating disorders, and personality disorders. Shedler came to three conclusions. First, psychodynamic therapies were as effective or more effective than CBT. Second, psychodynamic therapies resulted in an improvement maintained after the therapy ended. Third, the therapeutic relationship (involving transference phenomena and empathic attunement) is vital, as affirmed by subsequent research (Taylor 2012; Town et al. 2012). Shedler makes the striking point that incorporating psychodynamic techniques bolstered the effectiveness of other therapies.

I supervised a clinical psychologist (trained predominately in a CBT model) who wanted to find different ways of engaging with her clients. She said, while smiling impishly, 'Of course we work with the past, and transference, we've pinched all your best ideas'. Fonagy's (2015) meta-analysis identifies psychodynamic therapies to be effective, but not invariably so, for depression and some anxiety disorders, eating disorders, and somatic disorders. However, there is little evidence of effectiveness for post-traumatic stress disorder (PTSD), obsessive-compulsive disorder (OCD), bulimia, drug dependence, or psychotic conditions. The strongest evidence supports longer-term work with borderline personality disorder (BDP). Fonagy advocates adopting opportunities offered by bioscience and computational psychiatry that bridge neuroscience and clinical practice to 'creatively explore and assess the value of protocol-directed combinations of specific treatment components to address the key problems of individual patients' (2015: 137). Focusing on mentalisation-based therapy used in BDP, Bateman and Fonagy (2008, 2009) combined a long-term follow-up study and a RCT. This demonstrated the efficacy of dynamically informed mentalisation by identifying the quality of the relationship and a good working alliance as crucial for effectiveness. Dynamic therapies showed a lower relapse rate, with patients enjoying this approach but wanting more of it, for longer. Lilliengren and Sköndal's (2017) list of 200 RCTs involving psychodynamic approaches is an invaluable reference point that identifies the quality of the interactions in the therapist and the client as the most significant factor in resolving issues.

Summary

Research on the effectiveness of dynamic therapies is still in its infancy. It is hindered by a lack of central funding to develop the nuanced evidence base of psychoanalytic and psychodynamic practice-based evidence and contemporary quantitative analysis it requires, instead being dominated by a hierarchy of valuing research with RCTs at the pinnacle (Clarke 2018). Yakeley echoes this point, concluding:

> The provision of longer-term psychodynamic therapies is becoming increasingly scarce within the public sector, despite evidence that they may provide enduring positive outcomes in both symptom reduction and personality change. It remains our

responsibility to ensure that such evidence is fairly and openly communicated to commissioners and policy makers so that psychodynamic psychotherapies retain a legitimate place within the choice of evidence-based treatments available for our patients.

(2014: 277)

New research is always emerging that informs our therapeutic practice and helps our clients, so therapists should be research-active and engage with this vital area. We should also be aware of the on-going political battles about what constitutes research and what should be publicly funded, as it impacts not only on our practice but on the outcomes for our clients. Just as the research landscape is ever-changing, so too is the psychodynamic landscape, the focus of the next chapter.

Reflective questions

How does knowing about research supporting psychodynamic therapy influence your clinical practice or plans for clinical practice?

When did you last read a research paper, and how can you build this into your on-going development as a dynamic therapist?

4

Encountering the new – meeting a dancing landscape

This chapter examines why the term 'contemporary' in psychodynamic counselling and therapy means more than just new ideas. Underpinning therapy are important epistemic ideas about how we know and how we construct knowledge. The context of *contemporary* psychodynamic therapies draws from chaos and complexity theories and uses the analogies of fixed, rugged, and dancing landscapes. This chapter also considers how we can draw on the wisdom of the past and discover the energy of the new.

A shrine to the past

The whole purpose of therapy is to help the client, yet there is a danger that all therapies can become inward looking, serving their cherished traditions, beliefs, and practices, losing their dynamic presence. They become fixed in past patterns while our clients have embraced new ways of being that move and change like a dancing landscape. We will investigate this further later in this chapter.

Despite Freud's DNA being found in all dynamic therapies, we must avoid the danger of reifying the past, as if Freud were some nineteenth-century god to be worshipped in a present-day shrine. Neither should we ignore him just because some of his ideas have become superseded by new thinking and innovative research, or simply become unfashionable. A central psychodynamic idea is that the past influences the present and gaining insight into the past frees us to take new paths, paths not negotiated before. We can even be imprisoned by the past and make the same mistakes again and again. As Freud (1914b) memorably described it, it is a process of remembering (recalling the past), repeating (discovering the past in the therapy, through transference), and working through (finding new ways of relating to the past, with its significant figures) so we can become more fully alive, more fully ourselves.

Contemporary psychodynamic therapy

So what does contemporary psychodynamic therapy add to Freud? La Biennale di Venezia, established in 1896, is a prestigious international contemporary art exhibition that takes place from June to September on alternate years in Venice. Many of Britain's most famous (or infamous) artists and sculptors, such as Tracy Emin and Anthony Gormley, have represented Great Britain in what some have dubbed the art world's Olympics. Encountering cutting-edge art hosted in buildings spread across the whole of Venice is wondrous. Access is given to beautiful Grand Canal palazzos, back canal workshops, ancient churches, restored dockyards, and the purpose-built Biennale site where the new is juxtaposed with the old. The new and contemporary is set inside the old and mysterious, as if Venice itself becomes the art alongside its myths and mystique.

Contemporary psychodynamic therapy can be seen as a therapeutic equivalent of the Biennale. Its aim is to hold together the old and (re)discover the new, the radical, the cutting edge that has not yet become part of the popular therapeutic culture. In discovering the new, we can then see the old in a new light, as there are many insights still to be discovered in Freud. The intellectual basis for this is to be seen in the newly emerging thinking found in chaos and complexity theories. *Chaos* theory came initially from the natural sciences where it was observed that a very small change in a linear system could make the system behave differently, often in unexpected, unpredictable, and non-linear ways. *Complexity* theory developed out of chaos theory and focused on non-linear dynamics and their complex behaviours (or outcomes) due to the interactions of a large number of components. There is an inherent order in chaos theory (despite its name), while complexity theory operates on the edge of chaos, which is paradoxically both predictable and unpredictable. The terms chaos and complexity are sometimes subsumed under the single term, 'complexity'. The combination of the wisdom of the past and the vitality of the present are offered as a means to enable the reader to encounter contemporary psychodynamic therapy for themselves either as their central form of therapeutic practice or integrated into a wider range of therapeutic traditions. The challenge is to begin with the chaos of living now, in the real-world experience of our clients, and identify those minute changes that can profoundly influence a person's life. Reflect for a moment: what was your adolescence like? Through understanding the complex, multiple, overlapping psychodynamic perspectives that inform our thinking and practice, we can more fully engage with our clients on the edge of chaos about how to be fully human and how to come alive.

Jules' story

My friend Jules is a 35-year-old living in Manchester. She has a high-flying professional career but divorced when she was 30. Jules is vivacious and great fun to spend time with. She regales me with funny, sad, and poignant tales about on-line dating. Recently, she rang up to tell me she is in love, but he (in this case) doesn't seem to be taking her seriously. As I listened, it felt like she was 15, not 35. Should she call him, text him, email him – as she had not heard anything for 48 hours? Was she being too pushy? A litany of questions followed revealing anxieties about herself, her feelings, and whether she can risk trusting, with the potential for hurt or rejection. 'Who was she?' 'Was she attractive?' 'Was she too needy?' It emerged that at some point in the past, someone had said to her she was 'too clingy' and this had opened a wound that had never fully healed. As a friend, I simply listened and asked some questions, perhaps putting into words things Jules had not yet said but felt.

If Jules were a client, how would contemporary psychodynamic therapy help? This will become clear in later skills-led chapters, but is a reminder that therapy starts with the experience of the client in their world now, encountered in real-time therapeutic space. This enables a unique therapeutic encounter that starts from the here-and-now, and that can work forwards towards 'what-is-yet-to-be', and backwards to the 'there-and-then'. If we add in the idea that there is no time in the unconscious, as through the unconscious we can recall the distant past in the immediate present, especially in our feelings, this becomes a potent emotional cocktail. The fact that clients, through transference, can see us representing a wide range of people, or different characteristics of different people, all at the same time, throws us into the deep-end of another person's chaotic and complex psyche, as well as our own. Sometimes we struggle to swim in such tumultuous waters, yet being able to work with complex issues has always been one of the core appeals of psychoanalysis.

In the past, when faced with new complexities, the solution was to develop a single theoretical model that explained what was going on. Over time, one dominant psychoanalytic model became adopted, or replaced by another (see Chapter 5). The problem is that in swapping one kind of model – or theoretical system – for another, we repeat the limitations of the original linear model as it takes us along one clearly defined route. One of the crippling issues of Modernity (which formed the philosophical context of psychoanalysis) was that it privileged certain kinds of knowledge and neglected others. Postmodernity was a reaction to the failings of Modernity where every kind of knowledge became important and absolutes were rejected. If Modernity were parents, Postmodernity was the angry teenager that storms out of the house shouting, 'You don't understand. You always think you're right!' Contemporary psychodynamic therapy, too, is the teenager, now in their twenties or thirties, who can look back and think, 'I thought I knew everything. They (the parents) might have had a point'. Contemporary psychodynamic therapy offers the opportunity to work from multiple models and perspectives, neither rejecting the old, *classical* psychoanalysis, nor completely embracing every aspect of the new, *relational* psychoanalysis. It is not therefore simply a re-working of old ideas, passed down from one generation to another. It is the opportunity to develop something new, but in which elements of the past can clearly be seen. The philosophical basis for this can be found in the emergence of chaos and complexity theories as embryonic paradigms for therapy using the analogy of landscapes.

Complexity theory and the dancing landscape

Life is complex. My experience of working in a psychiatric hospital was formative at many levels. There on a ward, with the door often locked for safety, not security, I discovered the chaos that poor mental health brings. A world of delusions, conflicts, and tragedies, with patients often having the most profound insights into other patients, while remaining blind to their own conditions. It was a place of complexity, with no simple answers, where no sustainable linear arguments were convincing. Yet it was a touching place of human drama and encounter, shared laughter at the absurdity of life. On one occasion, in a group therapy session, a male patient, well-muscled and over 6 feet 4 inches tall, suddenly stood up and declared, 'I committed suicide once. I stepped in front of a bus, but I bounced off'. The rest of the group laughed at his unintended irony, as did he when he realised what he had said. My encounters in a psychiatric hospital taught me that life is complex, but also diminished if reduced to binary thinking or resorting to labels.

So why make psychodynamic therapies even more complex by introducing the ideas of complexity theory? Although Byrne applies complexity theory to the social sciences, arguing that 'linearity and order seemed . . . forced on the world which isn't really like that . . . There were flashes of light of the way to the sunrise of complexity theory' (1998: 3), we can see parallels with counselling or psychotherapy. It is these moments of illumination, which complexity theory can offer dynamic therapies, that makes it an intriguing area to explore as a recent entrant in the history of thought since the 1980s (Mitchell 2009). Rustin (2002) believes complexity theories offer something vital to psychoanalysis by embracing new transitions within, and creations of, new forms of knowledge. Complexity theory (an unpredictable development out of chaos theory) consists of a number of important ideas from various fields, including:

- life is complex, individually and collectively;
- we are all part of wider systems;
- systems are always in a process of adaptation, change, and growth;
- the greater the growth, the greater the complexity and the presence of unpredictability or chaos;
- the scientific ideas we normally use to understand such systems are often linear and predictable;
- such ideas do not help predict or deal with complexities and chaos, so new thinking is required; and
- new thinking enables us to deal with complexity, taking us to the edge of chaos, which is often where new developments are to be found.

The human being and their consciousness, which forms a unique self, is the most complex and chaotic system we will ever encounter. Our clients pour out stories of such agonising pain and bewildering complexity; they feel chaotic, not knowing what to do or where to go; disorder and confusion abound; we feel chaotic and look for guidance in our theoretical constructs, often finding them lacking. Page's (2010) landscape analogy identifies how we move from static systems of thinking to complex systems of thinking by identifying three types of landscapes where the optimal solution is to discover the peak in each one. Page writes from an evolutionary biological perspective but applies his ideas to business, economics, and politics, using the idea of fixed, rugged, and dancing landscapes. The landscape analogy offers a unique way of explaining contemporary developments in psychodynamic therapies.

A fixed landscape

In a fixed landscape model, there is a single mountain peak (Page uses Mount Fuji, Japan's highest mountain). This peak can be easily seen; there is an obvious trail to follow, which traverses upwards until you reach the summit. Fixed landscape thinking implies there is one summit, one route, and one form of accepted orthodoxy, most often linked to the linear, scientific thinking dominant in Modernity. Fixed landscape thinking dominated ideas in therapy for most of the twentieth century. Such thinking forms a reliable paradigm for understanding the way our minds work and how feelings and emotions emerge, and offers a route through the complex maze of the psyche. In the early 1960s, Kuhn (2012) developed the idea of paradigms where he observed we come to understand the world based on sets of inviolable assumptions that form the paradigm we live by. An example of a scientific paradigm can be seen in Freud's first women patients diagnosed with hysteria. Hysteria was believed to be excessive emotion and bizarre symptoms caused by problems in the uterus. Freud changed this paradigm by suggesting the causes lay in the psychological rather than the physical realm and even daring to say men could experience hysteria as well. Other forms of paradigms are social and cultural. They are a collection of unexamined assumptions, beliefs, and values we acquire and perceive to be the 'truth' or the 'right' thing to do. (My natural assumption is that it is best to drive on the right-hand side of the road but everyone in Europe disagrees with me!)

Yet paradigms change, change we resist, wedded as we are to old and comfortable ways of being. I possessed a pair of leather-soled brogues and, after years of use, they were moulded to my feet and felt delightfully comfortable. The problem? They leaked when it rained, resulting in damp socks. I could not bear to throw them away and kept them for 'dry use'. A time came, however, when they had to go and be replaced by new brogues, which proved to be lighter, just as comfortable, and waterproof – so I could use them all the time. We cannot bear to throw our 'leaky' paradigms away. We reify and feel comfortable in the past, and in a fixed landscape model stick to the one 'proper' route, rather than embrace alternative or newly emerging pathways. It is this underlying belief or tendency that results in the feuds that take place between different therapeutic traditions, and the hierarchical stance often found within psychodynamic therapies and discussions thereof. Sadly, I have often come across this when someone says, 'So you are *only* a counsellor', implying that they are superior in some way.

A rugged landscape

In a rugged landscape model, there are several mountains in a range with multiple peaks. Applied to psychoanalysis, this means that Jung or Lacan (whose ideas are very different from Freud's, even if they still value the unconscious) offer valuable ways of working with people's psyche. In counselling, we could point to Carl Rogers whose person-centred therapy is the very antithesis of Freud's psychoanalysis. If we adopted the previous strategy of following an obvious trail, we will find a peak, but not necessarily the peak we need, want, or that forms the summit. What is required is to explore the landscape first, following different trails and using the information obtained, before ascending the highest peak.

Consider the following analogy: whilst scrambling up the Three Sisters in Glencoe, we paused at what the GPS indicated was the highest point. Peering through the rain, others seemed higher. Clearly, our visual perspective was disorientated. It is challenging when hiking on a rugged landscape to gain a clear understanding of the nature of the landscape. What seems close can be exceedingly far, what appears easily navigable is in fact rather treacherous. A rugged landscape up close seems different from what is on the map. In such a rugged landscape, mountains are interconnected or intersected by cliff-faces, ridges, ravines, gorges, and valleys. Each offers a different perspective depending on what is required. For example, Ben Nevis is Britain's highest mountain and most people ascend it using the 'tourist' route. Yet, by far the most scenic and enjoyable route, if you like scrambling and have a head for heights, is the Càr Mòr Dearg ridge that curves round the back of Ben Nevis. This is not a route you find by accident. It is rarely busy and requires thought and preparation. Alternatively, there are routes that should only be tackled by a climber following careful observations of the foreboding rock face. What is important here is the value of exploring the trail before committing to a course of action in pursuit of a richly rewarding experience.

A dancing landscape

Finally, there is the dancing landscape, the importance of which is that it values emerging and collaborative processes. On the summits, and within the local peaks, gorges, and valleys, interdependent ecosystems emerge that offer new opportunities for development, not found in the other landscapes alone. These landscapes are dynamic and change with time, just as dancers move across the stage, combining form, structure, and spontaneity. In a dancing landscape, a greater level of exploration is required – and is encouraged – in order to discern the local peak and how this relates to other peaks, including the summit. Yet even when something is 'mapped', further time needs to be spent exploring what is on the verge of coming into view. Contemporary psychodynamic therapy invites you into a 'dancing' landscape and to take the risk of letting go the comfort of old paths and certainties found in 'fixed' or 'rugged' landscapes. But just as a long hard winter can enable a rock face to recover from the lichen-like environmental changes brought about by climate change's milder weather, a change in one part of the therapeutic and theoretical landscape influences other parts in ways that cannot easily be predicted.

Complexity theory and psychodynamic thought and practice

How does complexity theory and the analogy of alternative landscapes help us understand contemporary psychodynamic ideas? We have come a long way from Freud's original vision of psychoanalysis as a fixed landscape. Freud was the pioneer of a new conception of the unconscious, a new developmental psycho-biological theory, a new theory of the mind, as well as new therapeutic techniques. Without Freud's radical and fixed vision to reach the summit of the psyche, like the first ascent of Everest, we would be psychologically and therapeutically impoverished, as if gazing at the Himalayas from afar, dreaming that one day we could stand at the summit. The difficulty is that some seek a return to this fixed and single vision of psychoanalysis as an antidote to the complexity and chaos of contemporary life as presented by our clients. If challenged, they would deny this, but it is a driver of the conservatism of many psychoanalytic institutes and trainings (Kirsner 2000). If only it were that simple, limiting one's vision to a fixed landscape. Instead, in taking such an approach, we overlook the many other 'peaks' as the purity and simplicity does not fit with the lives of the clients we see. This nostalgic malaise pushes people to fit within a system, rather than engender a relationship that challenges our treasured thinking.

As seen in the rugged landscape model, new peaks with new vistas and opportunities emerged. While Everest is justly famous and the focus of much attention, more time is now being given to other peaks in the Khumba mountain range, of which Everest is a part. While Nuptse is only the twentieth highest, it is an alternative and, to some, no less-rewarding climb than Everest. It is a climb that might also offer a new perspective on its taller sister. Likewise, the rugged landscape of psychoanalysis evolved within itself as other peaks standing under the shadow of Freud slowly emerged.

Early key thinkers

While Freud excluded Jung, his ideas were still psychodynamic in principle and so Jung belongs as part of a psychodynamic rugged landscape (Papadopoulos 2006). Other early key thinkers and practitioners that emerged to refine or re-shape psychoanalysis, some of whom are explored in the Key Thinkers section, included Anna Freud (Midgley 2013), Ronald Fairbairn (Scharff and Scharff 2005), Melanie Klein (Likierman 2002), John Bowlby (Holmes 2014), Wilfred Bion (Mawson 2010), and Donald Winnicott (Abram 2013) in Britain; Heinz Hartmann (Schafer 1995) and Heinz Kohut (Siegel 1996; Mollon 2001) in the USA; and Jacques Lacan (Fink 1997) and Jean Laplanche (Scarfone 2013, 2015) in France.

It was never going to be easy to move from the dominance of a fixed landscape model, but the situation was not helped by Anna Freud and Melanie Klein's bloody civil war that broke out in the British Psychoanalytical Society between 1940 and 1943 (King and Steiner 1992). Others fared little better. Fairbairn remained ignored in splendid isolation in Scotland (Sutherland 1989). Bowlby developed attachment theory, which was viewed with suspicion as it was not a psychoanalytic theory of the mind. Bion, once seen as the heir to Klein's throne, moved to the liberating context of Los Angeles and his publications from this period became known as 'late Bion'. Some who value 'early Bion' are critical of his later work (Mawson 2010), while others find it immensely freeing (Eigen 1981; Grotstein 2007). Winnicott was viewed within the psychoanalytic establishment in Britain as a maverick figure (Kwawer 1998; Kahr 2016), who used novel ideas and unorthodox techniques. In the USA, Hartmann, with his colleagues Kris and Loewenstein, established a power base at the New York Psychoanalytic Society & Institute (NYPSI), which believed itself to be a defender of orthodox psychoanalysis (Kirsner 2000) – in essence, a return to a fixed landscape model. NYPSI re-shaped Freud's ideas as 'ego-psychology', which became the 'new orthodoxy', with only one official way to the summit. So when Kohut developed new psychoanalytic ideas, termed 'self-psychology', he was unsurprisingly marginalised by influential figures committed to classical psychoanalysis (Greenberg 2012).

In France, Lacan was highly critical of classical psychoanalysts arguing they had mis-read Freud. In taking such an iconoclastic stance, Lacan unconsciously set himself within the fixed landscape model, the very model he was trying to free people from. Laplanche, by con-trast, combined a closer reading of Freud with an extension into areas where Freud's thinking was more limited, including seduction theory, trauma, and gender (Fletcher 2013; Fletcher and Ray 2014; Scarfone 2015). Despite the resistances psychoanalysis encountered in the move from a fixed landscape to a rugged landscape, multiple forms of psychoanalytic think-ing and practice still survive. Many of the insights and techniques that shape the practice of psychoanalysis today inform my development of contemporary psychodynamic therapy.

Paradigm shifts

A contemporary psychodynamic approach offers a paradigm shift for psychodynamic and integrative therapies. The assumptions that form a paradigm serve well at the time but are often unhelpful in understanding new phenomena, as they tend to accommodate the new within existing structures – or ignore it as irrelevant. Kuhn argued there needed to be revo-lution, a paradigm shift, to understand new phenomena. People and institutions are heavily invested in old paradigms and resist the new. The evolution of the history of ideas is not one smooth linear rational advance in the pursuit of objective truth. Instead, it is one of radical disconcerting and subjective visions and counter-narratives that enable new truths to emerge and clash with the old. The move from a fixed to a rugged landscape accounts for the emerging complexity of psychoanalysis, psychiatry, psychotherapy, counselling, clinical psychology, and counselling psychology. These titles are still confusing to many people. Academic colleagues introduce me variously as a psychoanalyst, psychiatrist, psychologist, or psychotherapist, as if they are synonymous.

In Chapter 2, I offered a brief summary of how psychoanalysis, psychotherapy, counselling, and psychodynamic counselling emerged. When viewed through the lens of complexity theory, this can be understood as what happens when moving from a fixed to a rugged landscape model. The challenge facing all therapeutic traditions is to avoid returning to the security of a fixed landscape model, dominated by one peak, one exclusive way of understanding how human beings go wrong and how they can be helped. This is the philosophical flaw that underpins cognitive therapies (Gipps 2013). In trying to reduce people to cognitions, thought processes, and patterns, with symptom reduction as a common goal, this leaves significant dimensions of a person absent from the therapeutic process and relationship. The emergence of a rugged landscape model can be seen by the growth of integrative therapy since the 1980s. What makes an integrative approach different from an eclectic approach is an underlying philosophy of integration (Holmes and Bateman 2002; Hollanders 2007). Utilising the rugged and dancing landscape analogy of complexity theory can further enhance such a philosophy.

Lessons for the changing landscape

The role of diversity

The challenge facing therapists is that most of us have been trained in fixed or rugged landscape models, whereas our clients live in a dancing landscape. This is no easy task and is most often seen around issues of difference. A key change in the last twenty years, since the early 2000s, has been a much greater focus on issues of difference and diversity (Wheeler 2006). The central task for therapists working with individuals, couples, and groups, who form our societal fabric, is to address the profound issues of difference, diversity, and exclusion as they manifest not only in the clinical setting but in the day-to-day lives of our clients. Diversity is difficult to handle, as what makes us unique can also be what causes us rejection and shame. It is our uniqueness that calls for a radical engagement with the 'other', the person who is not me because otherness in a time of radical extremism, terrorist activity, and rampant race and gender issues is the challenge any form of therapy needs to face in order to address the needs of the future.

Ange's story

In her first session, Ange said 'I'm not sure why I am here'. She then burst into tears, which became convulsive sobbing. Her story tumbled out but became a sustained attack on herself and why she was never good enough. I found myself burning with shame that I knew didn't belong to me. What was it that Ange was so ashamed about? What was it that Ange was so split off from yet consumed her psyche? My intuition was to go slowly and allow Ange to tell me in her own time, as it felt like she could easily be shamed and, when we enter into our shame, it makes it difficult to think or feel anything else. Over the weeks, Ange told me of a cold, critical upbringing where she was clearly not regarded as important as her brothers. She always wanted to be a doctor but was told she was never going to be good enough, so 'why not be a nurse, as women are better at that'. 'Never good enough' became an internal monologue that seemed to grow in volume whenever she tried to achieve her goal. On the day she qualified as a doctor, instead of joy she felt despair that she did not know who she was. As therapy evolved around the issue of her identity, repairing damage done in her past, Ange voiced her shaming secret, 'I think I am gay'. She described herself as a reluctant lesbian, who in the following year began to value her uniqueness in an unashamed way. Ange discovered that she did not need to exist with a splintered psyche, shattered by shame, but could celebrate her uniqueness as wholly part of a beautiful emerging self.

At the heart of psychodynamic work is how we think about, and work with, diversity, an issue that forms a central task for all contemporary therapies (Wheeler 2006). We meet people as they are and help them discover the hidden, shame-inducing parts of themselves, forming these into a new part of their being.

Wisdom of the past and energy of the new

Contemporary psychodynamic therapy adopts values that support the vision to enter into the experience of the other by drawing on the wisdom of the past and energy of the new. Therapists have the opportunity to consider how these ideas about the other can be disseminated within the discipline of therapy and beyond. The value of complexity theory is that it allows for new connections (other than ones traditionally associated), and it is these new connections that bring diversity and life to existing systems of thought by offering new ways of viewing the core skills of psychotherapy. In real life, this is more challenging than you might think. We need a therapy that engages beyond the consulting room, the hermetically sealed bubble that protects the therapy from external intrusion. If we reach a consensus about the nature of the unconscious, expressed in the psyche in each of us, this dancing landscape is vitally present in any therapeutic space, whether we are therapist or patient.

Relationality as a way of being

Like a helicopter trip along the Grand Canyon, we have taken a scenic detour around the landscapes of psychodynamic therapies in the UK and beyond, in order to gain an understanding of where contemporary psychodynamic therapy locates itself. Centre-stage must be our clients because, as real people with real issues, they are at the heart of all psychodynamic therapies with the unique relationship that can be established. It is a relationship that changes the client and the therapist for the rest of our lives. Such a relationship requires moving into a dancing landscape where we are not quite sure what will emerge and where there is no one fixed way of being. Following in the line of thinking evolved by the writer and poet Nan Shepherd (1977, 2014), the intent is not that we conquer the summit of a new mountain called 'contemporary psychodynamic therapy', but that we enter into the mountain, journeying and discovering in ways that allow gentle transformations. This mountain is less a peak we conquer and more a place we inhabit.

Summary

A dancing landscape means we need to learn to dance as a therapist. Yet most of us need someone to show us the first steps, as we learn how to move in time with our own body and in partnership with another. In time, it becomes as natural as breathing. Being on the edge of chaos and complexity means we need to enter into an experience of our own aliveness that we can then offer to others. Therapy does not always give us the answers we want, and part of the therapeutic risk is to allow the questions to be asked while discovering enough of a sense of who we are. We help people to survive and thrive, to be able to make their own incomplete meaning. Such meaning enables the chaos to be experienced and, by facing the risk of stepping beyond our comfort zone or putting aside our defences, offers an opportunity to embrace being fully alive. This all happens because of a unique psychodynamic relationship.

I have adapted a landscape framework to understand how psychodynamic ideas have evolved into the forms we experience them today and how this reveals the opportunity for entering into the dancing landscape to discover for ourselves and our clients what we need for the future. A dancing landscape provides space for unique, local interactions to emerge that have not been seen elsewhere. So the form of psychotherapy that evolves in the UK will not be the same as that found in the USA, France, or South America, despite building on common theoretical foundations within each therapeutic tradition. By bringing together the complex system and the local interaction, new opportunities arise for unique forms of creativity and diversity (Page 2010).

The following chapters outline the steps we need to take in order to enable an effective psychodynamic therapeutic relationship to emerge and be sustained. Illustrating how we work with clients in a dancing landscape of therapy will be found later in the book once we have seen what features fit within this landscape. However, in the best Freudian tradition, we begin with the unconscious.

Reflective questions

Looking back on your training, or reflecting on your current training, what features of the different landscapes can you identify?

How do you believe our clients typically see us – fixed in the past or engaging with the new?

Looking at research

Although research in this area is in its infancy, the Society for Psychotherapy Research has launched a special interest group. Details are available at: https://www.psychotherapyresearch.org/page/CSiP [accessed 5 October 2018].

PART 2
Meeting the Unconscious

5

Who owns the unconscious?

Psychodynamic thought and practice has always been influenced by developments in psychoanalysis. But before going further, it will be helpful to say something about the scope of this chapter in order to avoid ambiguity or disappointment. A childhood memory to which we can all relate is a longed-for toy from Father Christmas. The excited, frantic unwrapping revealed all, only to be replaced by a growing unease on opening the box. The yearned-for 'Magic Set' bore little resemblance to the cheap plastic and paper-thin contents. There wasn't much magic, and all illusions were dispelled before you could say 'abracadabra' (much quicker than they are in therapy!). Still, your living room played host to many a magic show where you brought joy to your family with the flick of a wand. Similarly, while this chapter is not a detailed exposition of the major streams of psychoanalytic and psychodynamic thinking, it is a breathless and advantageous sprint around the psychodynamic block, trying to catch up with the fleeing unconscious, ever so close and yet so far away. The unconscious is the unique dimension of all psychodynamic therapies that marks them out as distinctive from other forms of therapy.

This chapter examines how Freud first understood the unconscious, set within the philosophical climate of his day. It then explores how, in the progression of psychoanalysis, our understanding of the unconscious has evolved into the multiple forms that exist today, replete with conflicts around the challenging question, 'Who owns the unconscious?' Freud's development of psychoanalysis significantly shaped the twentieth century in two particular ways. One was the idea of the unconscious defined as: the contents and mental states of the mind, just beyond the reach of conscious thought, but expressed through dreams and parapraxes (e.g. slips of the tongue, calling someone the wrong name, forgetting, leaving objects behind) in ways that influence our conscious behaviour and functioning. The other idea was the evolution of the self, especially the unconscious self, and the fascination with those aspects of the self that are beyond our control. We can know aspects of the unconscious after the event as we discern the impact on the self we are and want to become.

In the beginning . . .

My colleague Ali fixed her gaze on me across the restaurant table and stated, 'We cannot know the unconscious (pause) because it is unknowable' and laughed. This left me with a problem: 'How can I write a chapter about what is unknowable?' All I could do was write and see what emerged. It has often been assumed that the unconscious is the central unifying feature of all psychodynamic therapies. To offer multiple perspectives on the unconscious threatens to cut the tie that binds these traditions together. In line with chaos theory, out of this complexity comes new forms of creativity, and new opportunities to enter into the inner world – the dancing landscape – our clients inhabit.

A psychodynamic self

Mary's story

Mary was a client of mine who was very 'good': always on time, always said what she thought was the 'right' thing. Yet she was in therapy because she was stuck in her life, feeling she was going nowhere, not feeling anything 'real'. The language of emotions seemed alien to her. Her history was of fleeting relationships, each fading as she became hyper-critical of the other person. I was waiting for the moment when, through transference (see Chapters 7 and 13), I too became another figure (from her past, existing in her unconscious memory) that let her down. I did not have to wait long, though I cannot recall what triggered it. 'You're like all the rest', she shouted for the first time. 'Who have I just become for you?', I asked. She issued an expletive-ridden rant. Mary was so shocked at the words she'd just uttered, she instinctively put her hand over her mouth. It was too late. They were out there, echoing around the room, giving vent to an unexpected and unknown anger within. It transpired that she had been molested as a young teenager by an uncle who told her she was a 'bad' girl. Mary had spent the rest of her life trying to be a 'good' girl to prove to herself she wasn't bad, although that was how she still felt.

Like Mary, there comes a moment in life when we discover for the first time we don't understand ourselves. We do something 'out of character'. It is shocking because we also realise in that instant that it is a part of our character. We sense something different is motivating us when we realise there is a lust, a desire to possess, an anger, some hitherto unnoticed drive burning within. In short, we realise that the person we are is not the person we thought we were. This can come as a relief; at last, it makes sense of something that has been troubling us, something we suspected at some primitive level. Alternatively, it can arrive like a burglar, coming uninvited to steal our prized and hard-earned sense of self.

Welcome to the psychodynamic world, where these unknown aspects of who and what we are, the very 'self' we have become and are becoming, can be made sense of. In the twenty-first century, people go to therapists not just because something is troubling them, but because they are searching for some truth about themselves. They know it is 'out there', like aliens in 'The X-Files', but instead of scanning the skies, they search through fragmentary narratives and memories of a life lived, scanning the psyche for clues. Therapists try to make sense of who their clients are and how they have come to be the people they are in order to aid this complex process of self-discovery. People sometimes come to therapy not for a cure – although, if achievable, that is always helpful – but to make sense, to learn how to connect and relate, to find meaning, and to uncover hidden aspects of themselves. For contemporary psychodynamic therapists, unless we engage with the unconscious processes at work in us and our clients, somehow giving rise to the self that we have become, we are fumbling in the dark.

An essential dimension of a psychodynamic understanding of the 'self' is that it is irrepressibly dynamic. It may seem self-evident, but the 'self' is in a constant state of flux, evolving to the ever-changing circumstances, spiralling out in new trajectories. Think how one's sense of self and how one interacts with others is radically transformed by the beginning of a new career, the birth of a child, or a significant loss. Into every new situation, the psychodynamic 'self' brings its past and, in the present, the potential for new insights into aspects of our self comes into being. In contemporary psychodynamic counselling and therapy, we draw on our Freudian roots in making sense of our experiences through the idea of the unconscious.

The unconscious in the evolution of contemporary psychodynamic therapy

The unconscious is one of a handful of ideas that changed the world, forever. It was a paradigm shift, a revolution in thought intended to properly account for the observed phenomena. I once found my daughter, ever the curious and adventurous toddler, trying to insert one of my 12-inch vinyl records into a CD drive. She was frustrated it would not fit – the old and the new juxtaposed. My daughter is part of a generation when technology changed exponentially and altered our reference points. Like all paradigm shifts, it is difficult to imagine the world that went before. Likewise, it is unimaginable to perceive a world without reference to the idea of the unconscious. The notion of the unconscious is built into the foundation of all cultural thought in this century and the last, when Freud's *The Interpretation of Dreams* (1900) ushered in a new way of thinking.

There are various reasons why Freud's idea of the unconscious has had such a lasting impact. One of which is that the civilising veneer of the world we inhabited was ripped off, leaving a jagged hole lying just below the surface, when Freud opened up the uncomfortable truth of the human psyche for all to see. The term 'psyche', as we saw in Chapter 2, is used to refer to conscious and unconscious processes that fulfil or frustrate how we become a person in relation to ourselves and to others. The psyche helps us make sense of our drives towards creativity, destructiveness, and everything in between. By drawing attention within the psyche to the unconscious, we are able to examine the darker sides of human nature so brutally exposed in political upheaval and maltreatment of the 'other'. Psychodynamic thought helps us to understand the 'other' within, those parts of the self or psyche that are unknown, that we fear might be subversive, even dangerous. Focusing on the unconscious reveals what drives us, what we search and long for, what enables us to survive and thrive. The unconscious can also be the source of great creativity, releasing our energy and giving us life, freed from repression and restraint. Mark Rothko is one of my favourite artists. He believed his art was an expression of the unconscious allied to Greek tragedy that people could experience when they engaged with his large colourful canvases.

So the unconscious is a simple word but contains a vast galaxy of complex interlinked ideas and experiences. It is indisputably a part of us, a region of the mind that is unseen but acts in us and through us. It is, however, possible to view the unconscious from many different perspectives, each with areas that overlap as they dance across one another generating a plurality of meaning about the conscious and unconscious processes. Understanding more about the unconscious will inform and enrich our thinking and practice as dynamic or integrative therapists.

The philosophical context of the unconscious

Accounting for the origins and purpose of the unconscious stretches our thinking to its limits and strains language to the edge of comprehensibility. Can the nature of something we cannot see, or empirically prove, ever be described? Can something exist solely as a construct of the mind? Philosophers are still debating this – with some arguing for physicalism, which says that all mental things are in fact, in some sense, physical things while others posit such constructs of the mind as ontologically distinct things. (Through the centuries philosophical reflection on the unconscious has become increasingly sophisticated [Hendrix 2015].) By Freud's day, it was accepted that there were parts of the conscious mind that were not accessible but influenced people's actions. While Freud had trained as a neurologist, he was also widely read, versed in Greek literature and philosophy. His fascination with understanding the intricacies of human selfhood drove him on like an explorer of the new world (Schimmel 2014).

One of his key influences was Immanuel Kant, a prominent philosopher in the Enlightenment, the intellectual movement that emphasised reason and individualism. Kant developed the idea that the grounds for us believing in or knowing the self, for believing in or knowing an enduring mind, psyche, or subject unique to each of us and present throughout all of our lived experiences, are gained not from any *particular* experience but rather from the *nature and fact of* our experiences. For Kant, all experiences are characterised by a dynamic interplay whereby the self, as if by fixed and necessary laws, uniformly synthesises an apparent sensory input of raw data from the outside (or a collection of thoughts from the inside) in such a way that it grants spatiotemporal structure and causal order to this jumble of information – the self, so to speak, uniformly enables us to undergo meaningful and coherent experiences by bringing this collection of data into a structured whole. For instance, the self can bring together the various qualities of a clinical setting – the colour of the walls, the tone of the therapist's voice, the framed photograph on the side table – into a unified and orderly therapeutic encounter, an encounter we can comprehend as sequential events with causal links at a particular point in space and time: the therapist spoke to us in her Oxford-based room where she adjusted the photograph with the movement of her hand while sipping a coffee. Kant thus set up a conception of the self as involving a dynamic interplay in which it vitally influences how we undergo our day-to-day experiences. While we cannot, for Kant, know the self other than as an awareness of ourselves as the subject of certain experiences and beliefs, we can know how the self functions and have grounds for believing it to be there based on how things appear to us (as structured and orderly). If we consider this Kantian structuring self in parallel with Freud's unconscious-rich psyche, Kant can be seen as paving the way for us intuiting the dynamic boundaries of the conscious and unconscious mind and appreciating more fully the effects of the latter on the former – he provided grounds not only for us to believe in the unconscious but to be motivated to investigate how it is altering our lived worlds.

Another key philosophical context for the unconscious was Friedrich Nietzsche. Nietzsche believed that in all human behaviour, unconscious processes were at work that influenced our thoughts, feelings, memories, and actions. As he wrote in *The Gay Science* (1887):

> Man, like every living being, thinks continually without knowing it; thinking that rises to *consciousness* is only the smallest part of all this.
>
> (1887: 298)

He longed for a person to explore this, 'a philosophical *physician* in the exceptional sense of that word – one who has to pursue the problem of the total health of the people, time, race or of humanity' (1887: 35).

It was on Kant's foundational analysis of the self, and in accordance with Nietzsche's vision and habit of delving into the unseen drives behind our thoughts and actions, that Freud built his own ideas of the unconscious, and it was as a validation of these that Freud refers to Kant (Freud 1915b). One's experiences, for Kant, are always in part a product of one's self, they are always ordered and brought together by a self that we cannot directly experience but without which we could not make sense of or even undergo our experiences. Similarly, for Freud, the way we interact with the world is intimately related to our unconscious drives and, in a sense, is not possible without these drives – our unconscious drives make sense of and shape our conscious lives.

Freud devoted his attention to distinguishing conscious and unconscious processes in developing a new philosophy of the mind, and in this he was aware of another Enlightenment philosopher, G.W.F. Hegel, although he did not realise that Hegel, too, had developed ideas about the dynamic unconscious (Mills 2002). Hegel's ideas of 'thesis' and 'antithesis' engaged in a dialectic struggle captured the dynamic process of the unconscious in philosophical terms, although these concepts were more influential in Jung's thinking than Freud's (Solomon 1994). (The concept of a powerful dialectical process at work has also become significant in contemporary intersubjective and relational forms of psychoanalysis [Hoffman 1998, 2011].)

The importance of Enlightenment philosophy for Freud's understanding of the unconscious is to set it within a history of ideas of the mind that great thinkers had developed over the centuries. This does not detract from Freud's contribution, but rather sets the intellectual context for his quantum leap forward in our thinking about the unconscious.

Later in the century, Jacques Lacan's (see Key Thinkers) thinking – steeped as it was in both a radical new reading of Freud and (continental) philosophy – opened up new avenues of thought. An enigmatic figure, Lacan was part-philosopher, part-literary and cultural pioneer, and part-psychoanalyst who engaged with philosophy in innovative and creative ways (Kollias 2009). In the USA, Stolorow, Atwood, and Brandchaft evolved an intersubjective form of psychoanalysis that drew heavily on Heidegger, a key twentieth-century thinker, focusing on the essence of human existence (Atwood and Stolorow 1984; Orange et al. 1997). Building on this philosophical base, Orange (2010, 2011, 2016) integrates intersubjective thought, relational psychoanalysis, and self-psychology focused on what best helps people, with philosophy and the ethical imperative 'How shall we live?' at the centre of her work.

So philosophy and the unconscious are alive and well, offering new opportunities for enriching the work of dynamic and integrative therapists (Lear 2015). Yet we are jumping ahead, so here is a good point to return to Freud.

Freud's revolution and the unconscious

Freud was to change the way we think with his evolutionary and insightful theories of the psychological mind. Based on his Enlightenment roots, he believed that modern thinking needed to be freed from the constraints of metaphysics and religion, instead grounded in scientific ideas. Freud therefore inaugurated our understanding of the 'modern mind' that is still dominant today. Freud, Nietzsche's 'philosophical *physician*', took the ideas of the unconscious that already existed in Greek metaphysical and philosophical thought (Virgil, von Hartmann, Leibnitz, Herbart, Schopenhauer, and others), such as the restless underworld that could be stirred into life, and built them into a system rather than an abstract concept (Hendrix 2015). Freud's complex model of the mind synthesised existing ideas but he took them so much further than anyone before. Freud, his dreams, and the unconscious, were ready to be launched into the current century with the intent of rousing the world from its slumber.

Freud as a scientist believed that an explanation of human behaviour can be found by searching for a cause in the mental process of the individual's mind. It was what Freud did next, however, that makes him so unique. The mind, as elaborated by Freud, consisted of a unique amalgamation of philosophical, metaphysical, neurological, and psychological ideas, which he described through two models: the topographical and the structural.

Freud's topographical model

Freud first developed a vision of the mind that consisted of conscious, pre-conscious, and unconscious processes referred to as the topographical model (see Figure 5.1).

While people think of these processes as places, you cannot locate them in a region of the brain. They are instead language constructs used to describe a dynamic model of a mind. At its simplest, Freud's first model of the mind uses a spatial metaphor consisting of three layers. At the top there are the conscious aspects of the mind that rely on rational, logical thought that we are aware of (e.g. 'I am hungry and hot. I would like an ice-cream. I have money so I can go and buy one'). In the middle are the pre-conscious aspects of the

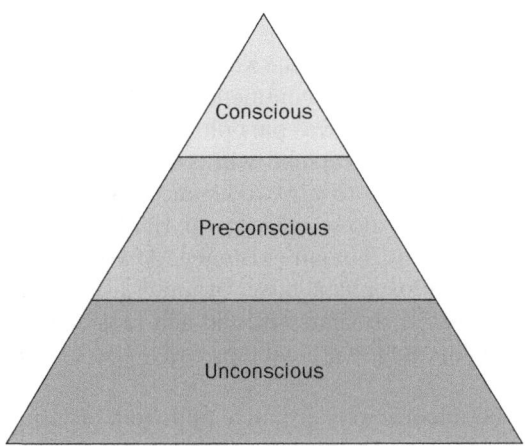

Figure 5.1 Topographical model

mind where desires and feelings from the unconscious begin to make themselves conscious, as in dreams (e.g. 'This weather reminds me of something I can't put into words, a sensation, a feeling, a dread', which emerges later that night in a dream of a childhood summer). As we get on with our daily lives, our conscious, waking life, teems with thoughts and feelings as we play it out – all the while, hovering in the wings, is the pre-conscious ready to make an entrance, as if we are on a theatre's centre stage. At the bottom is the unconscious. Sometimes referred to as the 'deep unconscious', this contains our most primitive, unbridled desires.

Why do you think our dreams can be so vibrant, violent, erotic, destructive, and confusing? Dreams are the royal route to the unconscious and give us disguised glimpses into a whole new universe contained within. This can be seen in Freud's case study based on his work with Sergei Pankejeff, who suffered from various phobias and obsessional traits. He became known as the 'Wolf Man' and he was seen initially by Freud from 1910 to 1914. Central to this analysis was the following dream: Pankejeff was lying on his bed one winter's night looking out of his window at a tree. The window suddenly flew open and he saw six or seven white wolves sitting in the branches of the tree. Terrified he was going to be eaten by the wolves, he screamed and woke up. Freud used free association with the 'Wolf Man' to uncover his associations of each component of the dream before Freud interpreted the terror of a young child encountering his parents having intercourse (the primal scene) and discovering his own sexuality. Pankejeff captured this powerful dream in a painting now displayed at the Freud Museum, London.

These are aspects of who we are expressed in thoughts, feelings, drives, and desires that have been driven from the conscious mind or repressed in some way. If these get out of kilter with one another, the result is anxiety (Freud 1910). Some thoughts are held back or down in a process of repression. Others are experienced as a gap or space where we know something should be but isn't. Repression does not work all the time. It is as if some parts of the unconscious are desperate for expression and so move into consciousness through the pre-conscious, with the pre-conscious acting like a Trojan horse. So the Freudian slip reveals hidden aspects of our inner self that have smuggled their way through the pre-conscious to arrive in consciousness.

Freud's structural model

Freud's understanding of the mind evolved through further reflections on his patients. In *The Ego and the Id* (1923), Freud re-shaped his thinking about the unconscious by developing a structural model utilising an anthropomorphic metaphor (Nettleton 2017). In Freud's new model, the id, ego, and super-ego jostle for position to most influence the psyche. Rather than being seen as abstract forces, they are better viewed as dynamic agencies acting as if they are 'persons' within us (see Figure 5.2).

Following his Darwin-influenced thinking, Freud believed human beings were driven by their instincts expressed as primitive somatic-based sexual and aggressive forces that stimulate all mental activity. This mental activity is captured by three terms: the id, the super-ego, and the ego, which form the psychic structure of the mind. The *id* is the unrestrained, seething, primitive part of us that seeks pleasure and knows no restraint but is repressed and always unconscious. The *super-ego* is the source of social, cultural, and religious beliefs, values, moral principles, and prohibitions. It draws on an internal world of significant figures in our life that influence our experience of ourselves through praise,

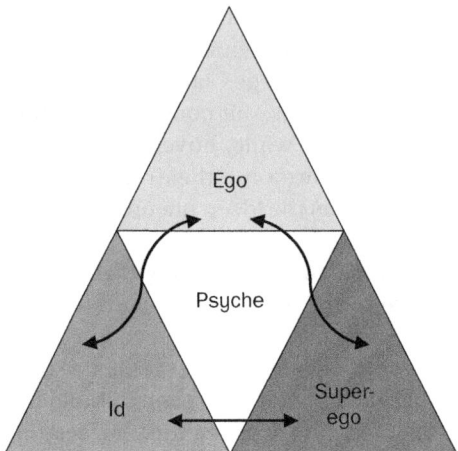

Figure 5.2 Structural model

punishment, judgement, criticism, restraint, and reward, and often operates to restrain the id. The *ego* balances the needs of the instincts, the external world, and the super-ego, existing in both the conscious and unconscious mind. These exist in a dynamic but delicate balance (as seen in the interconnected diagram), which can become unbalanced. Any model has its limitations and there is never a perfect balance. We can over-develop some aspects of the psyche: the super-ego drowns out our voice; the id overwhelms us with impulses or desires that cause havoc; and the ego can become overly rational in a way that robs us of that vital sense of aliveness mentioned in Chapter 4.

Combining the models

Freud distinguished these two models of the mind as adaptations of one another; yet, they are intimately connected and work together in a dynamic dance, weaving in and out of each other (Laplanche and Pontalis 1973). For example, in both Freud advocated unconscious processes as a way of understanding what it means to be human and as part of a psycho-biological system that accounts for human development and the growth of a person. A further commonality is that central to both of Freud's models of the mind is the role played by repression, which he viewed as one of the cornerstones of the whole structure of psychoanalysis (Freud 1914a, 1915a). Each person has an ability to regulate the experience of their emotions without fully knowing what they are doing. We are skilled at expelling from the conscious mind any powerful feeling that threatens to overwhelm us or that we find frightening or unpleasant. The opposite is also true – some feelings are so pleasurable we are afraid of them, tempting us like an alcoholic craving the next drink. Our mind banishes these feelings to some dark region inhabited by the unconscious.

So radical were Freud's ideas, and so powerful his clinical practices, that he captured the imagination of many who followed him (Gay 1998; Ross 2016b). While there were detractors, shocked at Freud's scandalous views about infantile sexuality, new analysts added their own clinical insights arising from observations of their patients. New ideas about the unconscious emerged, each claiming a unique place in psychoanalytic history.

Evolutions of the unconscious

As early as 1896, Freud wrote about a 'seduction hypothesis', which was that the hysterical symptoms he saw in adults were caused by the trauma of childhood sexual abuse. This convinced him about the power of the unconscious to keep secrets, but not forever. He later abandoned this theory when realising that many of these accounts of seduction were fantasised rather than real (although he never abandoned the view that in some patients actual abuse had occurred). This focused his thinking on the nature of wishes and fantasies, the origins of neuroses, and the power of the Oedipus myth. Freud saw the purpose of psychoanalysis as 'making conscious what has so far been unconscious' (1896: 164). However, he soon realised that uncovering the past, unconscious as it had been up until the moment of revelation, while cathartic for his patients, was not as therapeutically effective as he had assumed. He therefore re-evaluated the role of unconscious processes, replacing his initial 'seduction hypothesis' with a greater focus on the patient's intrapsychic world *and* unconscious processes. Freud used the term 'intrapsychic' to refer to being located in the mind of the person and often in conflict, as we saw in the relationships between the id, ego, and super-ego. The unconscious became the source from which all psychoanalytic and psychodynamic rivers flow and, like many rivers, there are multiple bends to navigate as the water contours through the landscape.

A brief history of the unconscious in psychoanalysis

We begin with a bird's eye view of the main developments in the history of psychoanalysis in relation to evolving understandings and uses of the unconscious. Such theoretical evolution is never a simple, straightforward, linear process. Instead, it is marked by profound disagreement and conflict, but knowing our feuding past can help us negotiate a more peaceful and productive future.

Freud and his early followers built on the idea of unconscious drives that shape us: a drive for survival of the species and a drive for the survival of the self. These drives were later configured to focus on sexuality (*eros*) and death (*thanatos*). Freud also used the term 'instincts' to refer to these unconscious drives. But overall, for Freud, how we develop requires a balancing act of what we need for survival and what we need for satisfaction. The two come into conflict, so we learn to repress these troubling demands coming from the unconscious. If that repression is too severe, it leads to an unease that can take the form of adult psychopathology.

Ian's story

Ian looked nervous, sitting uncomfortably on the settee. He told me he came to see me because a friend of his told him I had a 'Christian' background and so I would understand his problem. My immediate thought was that I was being labelled in some way in order to make Ian feel safe, which I heard as a form of unspoken communication saying, 'I don't feel safe'. He said he did not want to go to a 'non-Christian' psychiatrist as this might undermine his faith. I paradoxically thought that this was a defence against uncomfortable thoughts and feelings, and it is sadly true that some health professionals pathologise aspects of religious belief. I noticed I was experiencing a 'split' in my thinking, which left me wondering if this represented some aspect of Ian's yet-to-be-told story.

Ian explained he was from a Christian background that believed prayer and a greater degree of faith could cure emotional problems. These emotional problems were a product of how he perceived his sexuality, which he mumbled in an embarrassed way. Whilst occasionally sexually active with his wife, he kept having sexual thoughts about other women. The more he tried to supress these through reading his Bible and prayer, the worse they became. He avoided the computer because of the temptation to access pornography, which he felt would just make him feel guilty. (Freud, who championed a less inhibited sexual life, would have understood this as the part of the mind he termed the 'id' seeking satisfaction, and the 'super-ego' prohibiting this. The 'ego' was caught in-between and Ian's distress was experienced in forms of obsessional thoughts and overwhelming feelings of anxiety.)

We explored how he could engage in a conversation with his wife about sex, giving him and his wife the time and space to express what they wanted. We also touched on his nurturing mother and prohibitive father. In many ways, Ian typified a classical Oedipal dynamic (we will discuss this further in Chapter 8) but, in broaching the subject of sexuality, some prohibition was broken and matters resolved themselves. His obsessive thoughts receded (but never went away), and the symptoms of anxiety faded.

Much helpful psychodynamic therapy can happen in relatively few sessions where the past can be linked to the present whilst recognising a great deal more could be done in a longer therapeutic relationship. Ian had other issues that were clearly troubling him, not least his obsessional thinking, but his case illustrates how Freud's ideas are still relevant for understanding what goes on in us, consciously and unconsciously. Psychoanalysis has continually evolved, adopting different perspectives and elaborating distinctive aspects of the self, while retaining the core idea of the unconscious.

Warring mothers – Anna Freud and Klein

The feud between Freud and Jung (Falzeder 2012), which could have ripped apart the fabric of psychoanalysis, was nearly repeated thirty years later. Another Freud was involved, Anna, who, as explored in the previous chapter, was in a conflict with Melanie Klein (see Key Thinkers). Both child analysts, they had different theoretical understandings leading to impassioned discussions from 1941 to 1945 (King and Steiner 1992). Many Kleinian ideas are important for working as dynamic therapists (we shall explore these later), but at this stage, focusing on the unconscious, Klein and her followers offered invaluable new insights differing from those of Sigmund and Anna Freud. The unconscious in Klein operates from birth and consists of primitive states and the formation of various internal templates or prototypes that shape the emerging self. Klein's unconscious was a dark, symbolic place of deep passions, loves, hates, good breasts, bad breasts, part objects, biting, envy, jealousy, revenge, and annihilation. All this goes on in the infant's mind from day one as it is consumed by instinctive passions, biologically driven for surviving and searching for the best object to provide for its needs, so engaging with children in their play was crucial as it made a child's most primitive unconscious aspects become accessible to the analyst. Klein invented a word to describe this alien landscape and these complex processes: all this occurs in the mind in the form of 'phantasy', which stressed the unconscious nature of these experiences. Klein's aim was to find a way of constructing a meaningful narrative based on early emotional experiences that tell the story of our internal world dichotomies: pleasure and pain; love and hate; and good and bad.

Some think Anna Freud was wrong to ignore these primitive unconscious aspects found in a child's play, rather seeing them as a royal route to the child's unconscious processes (Likierman 2002). Kleinian and post-Kleinian ideas became the dominant – but not the only – tradition in British psychoanalysis, child analysis, and psychotherapy (Rustin and Rustin 2016). The work of Fairbairn (Sutherland 1989; Scharff and Scharff 2005), Guntrip (Hazell 1996), Balint (Stewart 1996), Bowlby (see Key Thinkers; Coates 2004), and Winnicott (Abram 2013) formed the British Object Relations School, the 'Independents' or the 'Middle Group' who were neither aligned with Klein nor Anna Freud (Kohon 1986). Other key figures included Sharpe, Brierley, Payne, Heimann, Kahn, Ryecroft, and Foulkes (Rayner 1991). Unlike other psychoanalytic tributaries, this formed a broad delta with many streams converging while maintaining a unity around the nature of the unconscious.

Good-enough mothers – Winnicott

The best-known and most distinctive ideas of the 'Independents' came from Donald Winnicott. Throughout his life, Winnicott maintained his clinical practice as a paediatrician, which grounded his theories in lived experience. Winnicott's understanding of the unconscious has been overlooked but is now being re-appraised and shown to value creativity, paradox, and dialectic thought that emerges through the unconscious to become present in the therapeutic space (Widlöcher 2013). According to Ogden (2013), a contemporary American psychoanalyst influenced by Klein and Winnicott, the unconscious mind and the evolution of the conscious mind come into being and work together when a baby discovers two different kinds of experience arising from the same psychological event. So a baby can love and hate at the same time; they can be dependent and omnipotent; they can be separate and joined, with the conscious and unconscious mind allowing the baby to experience its own unique sense of being. This includes incorporating a true self and multiple false selves (see Chapter 13). The baby's internal world requires a mother or carer to enable this, hence Winnicott's view of the mother or carer as the 'facilitating environment'. For Winnicott, it was impossible to talk about a baby without talking about a mother. The paradox is the baby is both the object and the environment, and mother the environment and the object (Winnicott 2013). For Winnicott, the unconscious functioned less as the vehicle and container for the satisfaction of drives, as found in Freud, and more as a dyadic context for the emergence of being (Loparic 2013). As Winnicott said, there is no such thing as *a baby*. There is always *a baby and a mother*, or carer, who brings the psychological life of the baby into being through their gaze, touch, holding, and other interactions (see Chapter 9).

Persecution and promise – Europe and the USA

Ego psychology

The Nazi persecution of Jews and Jewish psychoanalysts (a few non-Jewish psychoanalysts remained in Germany) led to a rapid dispersal of Jewish psychoanalysts around the world, especially the USA. Karen Horney arrived in New York in 1930, searching for a freer psychoanalytic context in which to do new thinking. As the Nazi Party gained power and influence, the exodus of psychoanalysts to the USA included Fromm (1934), Erikson (1935), Fenichel (1938), Kris (1940), Hartmann (1941), and Loewenstein (1942), amongst others. The latter three, based in New York, built on Sigmund and Anna Freud's ideas, developing a new emphasis termed 'ego psychology'. Loewenstein had been in analysis with Freud and was seen by some as an heir to Freud in this new American context. Taking Freud's structural model, utilising Anna Freud's (1936) work on the defences, and building on Hartmann's work on ego adaptation (1958), ego psychology gave the ego a more prominent role in the psyche, seeing it as relatively independent from the unconscious demands of the id and the super-ego. While the unconscious was still crucially important, it was viewed as designed to seek adaptation to the environment and aid ego adaptation rather than remaining a kind of pleasure-seeking baby wishing to satisfy its drives.

Self-psychology

Ego psychology's focus on the ego as balancing unconscious and environmental factors was challenged by a new emphasis on the 'self' as the central focus of psychoanalytic reflection, through the work of Kohut and 'self-psychology' (Mollon 2001; Strozier 2001). Described as 'revolutionary', it breathed new life into American psychoanalysis. Kohut's view of the unconscious was that the impulses and conflicts it contained acted as psychic defences against the unspeakable dread of 'disintegration'. This is the overwhelming feeling of extreme anxiety a person feels associated with the sense of falling to pieces, and a fear they can never be re-connected or repaired. Kohut's ideas capture our deepest anxiety and echo Bion's idea of 'nameless dread', where a mother is unable to contain or transform a baby's deepest fears, leaving the baby with the feeling it is dying, experiencing a dread with life stripped of meaning. Like Grotstein (Ross and Loly 2013), Mollon uses the analogy of an astronomical black hole to explore Kohut's unconscious:

> [In the unconscious is an absence,] a hole where the core self should be . . . analogous to an astronomical black hole, invisible and discernible only through its secondary effects . . . psychodynamic conflict is used itself as a defence against the deeper danger – the breakup of the self . . . Thus the fundamental danger is of fragmentation . . . it is as if Kohut began to look beyond the visible and manifest (albeit unconscious) realms of the psyche and found the areas of dark matter and black holes that account for what is observed. The selfobject transferences, of mirroring, idealising and twinship, tend to be invisible until they are disrupted. It is through the breakdown products of their destruction that their existence is discerned.
>
> (Mollon 2016)

Kohut shifted the focus from the presence of the unconscious as the driving force to the emergence of the self, navigating through conscious and unconscious processes. In doing so, Kohut enabled psychoanalysis to engage with one of the most pressing problems of our time, narcissism.

The French Revolution – Jacques Lacan

Just as Kohut advanced a new shape to the unconscious in a North American context, in Europe a radical French psychoanalytic thinker materialised in Jacques Lacan. Writing before Kohut, Lacan argued that the unconscious was structured like a language, an idea that took root in analytic, literary, sociological, philosophical, and cultural studies. Unlike Freud, Lacan saw a baby as having no unconscious riven with drives – neither physical nor emotional. Rather, a baby has an unconscious expressed in a potential for thinking.

In Fink (1997, 2017) and Bailly's (2009) expositions and critiques of Lacan's elusive thinking, a unique view of the unconscious emerges. In Freud, everything flows from the unconscious. For Lacan, the unconscious was a strange, elusive idea that we become curious about and want to work out what it means. The unconscious was here a later development, of importance because it forms the location of proto-thinking, containing concepts and hypotheses based on the earliest embodied experiences with a mother. This enables the idea of a mother to become a signifier in the mind of the baby and therefore able to be part of a discourse. There also exists a silent proto-language, as yet unspoken, that as the baby begins to gather its thoughts and put them into language enables the discovery of the unconscious. As Lacan famously said, the unconscious is structured like a language with a capacity to invent, signify, speak, and enter into discourse – the unconscious is the discourse of the Other, connecting us within ourselves and to others. The unconscious contains many signifiers linked in chains of thought, like a stream of consciousness or, in this case, a stream of *unconsciousness*. Lacan's ideas regarding the unconscious are an important contribution to contemporary psychoanalysis and one key to unlocking his notoriously complex thinking for contemporary psychodynamic therapy.

Ian's story re-visited

Returning to Ian (who was struggling with sexuality), how might these different understandings of the unconscious shape the process of therapy?

From a Kleinian perspective, Ian's psychic defence is 'splitting' and he is located in a paranoid-schizoid position, caught up in a struggle between good and bad: legitimate sexual thoughts about his wife versus lustful thoughts about other women; Christian thoughts, beliefs, and actions, such as praying versus the lure of pornography and guilt; a longing for intimacy versus a fear of women (etc.). He also uses idealisation as a defence (i.e. a Christian therapist can help him much more than a secular psychiatrist). It would appear there are plenty of persecutory objects in Ian's internal world and persecutory anxieties in his external world that need to be recognised before moving to a depressive position.

From a Kohutian perspective, Ian's unconscious need is for a good experience of narcissism, of being loved, wanted, and desired by a mother and a father – as well as a wife. In their felt absence, he projects his needs onto others, whereas he needs to discover this within himself.

From a Lacanian perspective, not only is the unconscious structured like a language, Lacan found the key to Freudian unconscious as a chain of signifiers. Close attention would be paid to Ian's language and the layers of symbolism attached to this expressing, as it would, aspects of unconscious thoughts, feelings, and desires. This could include identifying what the chain or links were and what these signified in his unconscious.

Summary

Having taken you on a fast route march up a steep highland path of nineteenth-, twentieth-, and twenty-first-century thought related to psychoanalysis, we can now pause, get our breath back, fill our lungs with clear mountain air, and ask the question: 'Why is it important to understand these evolutionary stages in the development of the unconscious?'

As we move into a dancing landscape of dynamic therapy, we are enriched by multiple understandings of the unconscious and are not limited to any one approach. In the case of Ian, each expression of the unconscious could result in creative and effective therapy. The unconscious is such a powerful idea, and paradoxically still knowingly unknowable, that other forms, understandings, and expressions of the unconscious have emerged that are now part of an exciting, evolving, and unpredictable landscape, as we shall see in the next chapter.

Reflective questions

Which of the thinkers discussed in this chapter best inform your *understanding of* the unconscious?

Of the theories examined, which *intuitively connects* with you?

Using Freud's categories of id, ego, and super-ego, reflect on your clinical work or the cases you have read about. How have they been evidenced?

Looking at research

Bargh, J. and Morsella, E. (2008) The unconscious mind, *Perspectives on Psychological Science*, 3(1): 73–79.

6

The evolving unconscious

This chapter explores the multiple forms and understandings of the unconscious that illuminate our understanding of what is going on in us and our clients. This knowledge has the potential to transform our practice as psychodynamic or integrative practitioners. These multiple expressions include: the collective and mythological unconscious; the creative unconscious in its many aesthetic, numinous, and mystical forms; the intersubjective unconscious; neuroscience and the unconscious; concluding with the social unconscious. Each variety of the unconscious has the opportunity to move across your mind as you engage with each, separately and together, forming a new encounter with the unconscious.

A spiritual psyche – Jung's collective and mythological unconscious

Carl Jung (see Key Thinkers) developed distinctive ideas about the unconscious that went beyond the limitations he saw in Freud's scientific thought. Jung reached back in time and offered a view of the *collective* unconscious, by which he meant an objective, non-personal psychic inheritance that acts as a repository of ideas and images linked to his idea of archetypes as universal symbolic figures. The collective unconscious is thus the potential psychic legacy of humankind, which lays below the *personal* unconscious of Freud (Shamdasani 2003).

Their difference becomes most apparent on the subject of dreams. Falzeder compares the science of Freud with the art of Jung. Freud used a scientific analogy of breaking down complex substances to basic elements; Jung saw dreams as raw, spontaneous products of the unconscious expressing the 'unitary soul of humanity' that should not be analysed. As he wrote, 'They are pure nature; they show us the unvarnished, natural truth' (Jung 1933: 317). They consist of living symbols that offer meaning through the use of an active imagining utilising 'amplification' that finds counterparts 'to those images in "collective" imaginations, such as myths, religious systems and practices, visions, alchemy, yoga, and so on' (Falzeder 2012: 27f.). Falzeder's insight reveals the deep tensions that lay between Freud and Jung. Sayers (2003) identifies another difference, one related to God. What Freud saw as 'illusion', Jung discussed as 'encounter'. For Jung, it is in the unconscious that we encounter a oneness with God that brings therapeutic benefit. The unconscious is here inclusive and collective, incorporating that which is beyond. A similarly inclusive understanding is found in popular culture where the collective unconscious is an idea that has a rich currency. Jung saw the collective unconscious as deeper, richer, and less trauma-driven than Freud's unconscious, finding evidence in myths, fairy-stories, religious texts, symbols, and rituals that made sense of human experiences and supported Jung's spiritual view of the self.

Jungian psychology and Freudian psychoanalysis were to go their separate ways, like the two brothers in the 'Prodigal Son' (Luke 15; Nouwen 1992). Jung was rather more forgiving and offered a token of 'return' by sending a patient to Freud in 1923. It was their shared belief in the unconscious that had brought Freud and Jung together, and it was their different perspectives on the unconscious that shattered this early bond and deprived psychoanalysis of a creative dialogue.

As Jungian psychology has evolved, there is a specific focus on the unconscious structured as a myth, or myths, unlike the single defining myth of Oedipus beloved by Freud (Adams 2010), which we will explore in the following chapter. In working with the unconscious, Adams finds support in the ideas of Bion, who sees value in working clinically with myths as a way of understanding early relationships, especially with parents. Only now are the two traditions finding a rapprochement, primarily through relational psychoanalysis (Eigen 1998). This is vitally important, as the understanding of the unconscious that many of our clients bring into the therapeutic space includes a 'collective' dimension. To them, it makes sense and is implicit in much of their thinking and sense-making. It is waiting like some dormant archetypal dragon to be roused from slumber and breathe fire into so many forms of creativity.

The creative unconscious

There are dimensions to the unconscious that people have tried to capture with terms like 'aesthetic', 'mystical', 'numinous', and 'mnemic'. All are creative in intent. They result in something that originates in, or is experienced through, the unconscious, something that cannot be fully captured in words. Yet words are all we have and we use them in order to catch fleeting glimpses of things we sense deeply. Many writers attribute the unconscious as the location of their creativity or tie the creativity they perceive in the writings of others to the unconscious aspects of the author. This creativity can be a desire to recover something seen as important, but not yet known, part of the past, individually or collectively, that has been lost in time but is waiting to be found. Jacqueline Rose, writing about Virginia Woolf, refers to the unconscious knowing something more profoundly than conscious thought:

> Once you introduce the unconscious into the frame . . . then it becomes impossible, . . . to regulate the forms of traffic between present, future and past, between the living and the dead. To be a subject [is to] be haunted . . . being haunted, might indeed be another word for writing.
>
> (2003: 87)

The haunting images found in surrealist art accord with Rose's intuitions about Woolf. Surrealism as an avant-garde art movement began in Paris in the 1920s and located the modern man or woman in the centre of the forces unleashed by the unconscious, most often encountered in dreams or symbols. Its aim was to reveal the unconscious and reconcile it with rational life. For example, Dalí's paintings combine symbols and the surreal, just as one encounters in dreams taken to analysts for interpretation. By the 1940s, the surrealist idea of revealing the unconscious influenced the new art movement of abstract expressionism. Rothko, Pollock, de Kooning, and others sought to express the uncon-scious through abstraction using new, spontaneous techniques rather than dream-like objects or images. Many of their pictures when encountered pulse with life and stir something within, as if the unconscious of the artist still engages with the unconscious of the viewer (Sayers 2007).

Christopher Bollas, a contemporary psychoanalyst and writer, in discussing de Kooning admires how the unconscious comes through the painting, with multiple layers of paint being scraped away, lines being painted over, with something appearing beneath the sur-face as the artistic vision is worked and re-worked. This expresses the creative dynamics found in the unconscious (Molino 1997). Bollas' work is steeped in the ideas of Winnicott and Bion, as well as French psychoanalysis, and he offers a creative understanding of psy-choanalysis that has its origin in his new understanding of the unconscious (Scalia 2002; Nettleton 2017). Bollas viewed Freud's vision of the unconscious as the repressed uncon-scious (1989) and, while original in its time, Bollas argues this fails to pursue other aspects of unconscious perception, unconscious communication, and unconscious creativity, found in Freud's thinking only in embryonic form. He proposed a new model of the mind allying the repressed unconscious with a receptive or received unconscious. The mind is relent-lessly creative, developing new links, making connections, forming images, thoughts, and associations in an alive place that is chaotic and complex. These connections are ready to be called into action and are most clearly seen in the process of dreaming, where the uncon-scious combines the stored data with the new psychically rich data of the past day. For Bollas,

> [A dream] is not only a remarkable aesthetic accomplishment, it is the most sophisti-cated thinking we have. A dream can think thousands of thoughts in a few seconds, its sheer efficiency is breathtaking. It can present past, present, and imagined future in one single image.
>
> (2007: 72f.)

Each person's unconscious is unique and creative, seeking to express the subject's 'idiom', as Bollas terms it, as a way of being and a reaching towards their true self. This is not some pre-defined template, rather a unique range of possibilities that emerges within each person as they seek their true self (Bollas 1987). Building on this, Bollas evolved the idea of an 'unthought known', something an adult knows without thinking about how they know it, that exists in the infant's unconscious based on our earliest relational experiences, which becomes registered in the psyche, often in symbolic form, before language.

Jane's story

Jane came for therapy because she felt people always let her down. Arranging therapy was difficult because she had a young baby who was very demanding, and Jane in turn was very demanding with me. At some stage, I suggested that she bring her *internal* 'young baby' into the room.

As she told her story, Jane 'remembered' that her mother told her she was always a difficult baby and that she could never give her enough milk. Behind this verbal remembering lies Jane's 'unthought known': she was a greedy baby and never satisfied, a pattern she replicated in her relationships. Jane 'knew' this because it was fundamental to her being; the mother who couldn't manage her baby's neediness had instilled in her, as a 'transformational object', a sense of herself as too much, too demanding, so her expectation was that she would be let down – because she was. Her needs were too much and no one could meet them. The reason she was in therapy was because it wasn't known consciously and it was only when she was able to get in touch with her very early infant self that her relational dynamic began to make sense.

Unthought knowns form the foundations of who the person is to become yet wait passively to be discovered in new and creative ways. The self of the baby and the maternal object interact in a two-way process drawing on the presence of unconscious aspects of the unthought known. The mother has the potential to become a transformational object providing an 'aesthetic moment'. The baby discovers it is good to be alive, to be creative, to risk and trust. Psychodynamic therapies offer each person the opportunity to (re-)discover such transformations or aesthetic moments in working with the creative, receptive unconscious in all its complexity (Bollas 2009; Nettleton 2017).

The numinous unconscious

Accepting the unconscious as a sphere of human experience that cannot be fully known or put into words, this takes us back to the very beginning and has direct parallels with numinous or mystical experiences. While we try and capture these experiences in words, something is always lost in translation. We may remember the time and the place but the actual experience itself is elusive and we struggle to communicate this to others. We work with fleeting images, feelings, and the ghosts of memories that Freud thought of as memory traces or mnemic symbols (1900) to convey the unconveyable. The depths of such experiences elude our ability to recall immediately but with a knowing on our part that they reside in the unconscious, waiting to be recalled by a word, a sound, an image, a smell, or a sensation. This links with Bion's concept of 'O', as he strains the limits of language to express what he viewed as 'ultimate reality' or 'absolute truth', which like the unconscious he viewed as unknown and unknowable. In therapy, some clients claim to encounter an at-oneness with O or a higher, ultimate reality, in some sense, through openness to what is unknown or unknowable, which takes us into the realms of the numinous and the mystical. For them, this becomes a transforming experience.

Two contemporary psychoanalysts, Grotstein (2007) and Eigen (1981, 1998, 2012, 2014), have taken up this concept of O. While forms of religious, spiritual, or sacred language are generally excluded from psychoanalysis (Kenny 2015), this overlooked expression of the unconscious continues to surface throughout the history of psychoanalysis (Ross 2010).

While we have examined creative, aesthetic, numinous, and mystical expressions of the unconscious, the therapeutic encounter is ultimately about two people meeting. Just as a writer needs a reader, a therapist needs a client in bringing to life something unique that happens between two people. The term used to account for this is 'intersubjectivity'.

The intersubjective and relational unconscious

The term 'intersubjectivity' brings together more than one subjectivity, a dynamic found in all relationships. Atwood and Stolorow (1984) and colleagues applied this thinking to psychoanalysis, advancing the idea of three inter-related, intersubjectively derived forms of the unconscious:

- the *pre-reflective*: processes that are out of our focus or awareness but that still influence us;
- the *dynamic*, with a fluid boundary between conscious and unconscious affect states; and
- the *unvalidated*: experiences we are not able to put into words yet exist without evoking any form of validation.

Recurring patterns of intersubjective, feeling-laden transactions and relationships, conscious and unconscious, are typically established between mother and baby, and these become unconsciously repeated patterns in subsequent relationships. This approach takes ideas from past figures, such as Ferenczi and Sullivan, and allies them to emerging ideas (Spezzano 2012) illustrating how a dancing landscape of dynamic theory and practice offers us something creative and new that could not have been foreseen.

Intersubjectivity in contemporary psychodynamic therapy

An analogy might help illustrate what this means. Having taught myself to play squash, it became clear when playing others that most, if not all, of my technique was very poor. What I made up for in youthful effort could not be covered over when playing a skilful opponent, or when that youthful energy ran out. The partner of a colleague offered to coach me. It meant dismantling before re-assembling. It was painful to experience, but what made all the difference was that he did far more than observe – he also played squash with me. Seeing someone else on the court enabled a different experience. He had to run, sweat, stretch, and strain. He missed serves. He was playing in a very real way while teaching me. I was touched by his belief in me – it enabled me to move to the next stage. This is analogous to the intersubjective approach to psychodynamic therapy. In the consulting room, there are two subjectivities that interact with each other. One of these persons is termed 'analyst', 'therapist', or 'counsellor', terms loaded with a particular knowledge and experience, and the other is termed 'analysand', 'patient', or 'client'. What proves to be therapeutic is the engagement of the two subjectivities in the therapeutic space, intermingling, enacting, and mutually transforming. This happens at both a conscious and an unconscious level. There are two unconsciousnesses at work.

Intersubjectivity, and the intersubjective unconscious, have a different philosophical base from Freud's unconscious, rooted as it is in the phenomenology of Husserl, Heidegger, and the like. Such an intersubjective approach is closely related to the idea of the *relational* unconscious. When two unconscious minds come together, they have a reciprocal influence that creates a relational unconscious, which goes beyond each individual's conscious and unconscious being. So,

> the relational unconscious is the unrecognized bond that wraps each relationship, infusing the expression and constriction of each partner's subjectivity and individual unconscious within that particular relation . . . the relational unconscious is a concept

that allows the joining of psychoanalytic thought about intrapsychic and intersubjective phenomena within a theoretical framework that contains each perspective and elaborates their inherent interconnectedness.

(Gerson 2004: 71f.)

The relational unconscious exists and is waiting to be discovered in the psyche of two people that meet. The relationship is the vehicle for therapeutic discovery where both parties find transformative intersubjective insight; however, a therapeutic relationship needs to provide safe boundaries in which transformation happens. While aspects of the unconscious are unknowable, something happens in a 'two' that does not happen when being a 'one'. Uncovering the details of intersubjective processes includes what occurs in the brain, and what occurs in the wider group at a social level. At the very least, neuroscience and its application to psychoanalysis – neuropsychoanalysis – supports the idea of unconscious processing and, as Solms (1997, 2013) argues convincingly, validates psychodynamic thinking (see Chapter 10).

The social unconscious

Jung's collective unconscious points to something beyond the individual, reaching back into the past and remaining as symbols, or archetypes, to be encountered in the present. A parallel idea emerged through the work of Foulkes, who had worked briefly with Jung in his early days. Foulkes developed the idea of the 'social unconscious', the origins of which are found in his *Therapeutic Group Analysis* (1964). The term 'social unconscious' refers to social, cultural, beliefs, values, and forms of communication that are beyond conscious awareness yet shape the society of which we are part. Weinberg (2007) adapts Foulkes' thinking about the social dimension of a group to include the following four levels: the current, transferential, projective, and primordial. Psychodynamic therapists are familiar with: the *current*, the here-and-now experiences we encounter in groups; the *transferential*, the seeing others in groups as if they were significant figures from our past; and the *projective*, putting our unwanted or uncomfortable thoughts, feelings, and emotions into another person or group. What may be new is the primordial level, referring to Jungian ideas of myths, archetypes, and other aspects of the collective unconscious. Having established the shape of the group unconscious, Foulkes believes a foundation matrix consisting of shared anxieties and fantasies links each group and larger social groups.

Building on this foundation emerges the idea of the social or interpersonal unconscious. Hopper (1996, 2001, 2003) and Dalal (1998, 2011) have developed this concept in different but parallel ways, thus enlarging the scope of how the social unconscious impacts at all levels, how the social structures can shape the unconscious, as well as addressing issues of power. The social unconscious is a co-constructed unconscious drawn from communities, societies, nations, and cultures. It consists of shared anxieties, fears, traumas, fantasies, defences, myths, and memories. It challenges the unspoken power dynamics to be found in all groups. Clients come with an entire history stretching back generations, often traumatic, that needs a space to be re-visited. This often features in psychodynamic work with asylum-seekers and refugees who bring the traumas that led them to flee their home, and the trauma of travelling to, and being in, a new country. If we are able to offer time and space for this social unconscious to find a life, hungry ghosts can become treasured ancestors (Mitchell 1998). Like our clients, each of us has our own social unconscious – and we ignore this at our peril.

Our evolving unconscious

Our exploration of the unconscious so far has left unanswered several vital questions, including:

- Are all expressions of the unconscious equal?
- Does each offer the same therapeutic value and deserve equal attention?

It is my conviction we can best help our clients by finding a way of working with multiple forms of the unconscious. To limit oneself to a single view of the unconscious limits the richness, depth, and creativity possible in engaging with unconscious experience, as there is not one 'truth' about the unconscious. No single view of the unconscious triumphs over all others, as Freud thought. Yet for psychodynamic therapists and integrative therapists using psychodynamic ideas, working with the unconscious is always about a third dimension, a waiting, brooding presence, pregnant, waiting for a time to be born. It is an 'unthought known', as Bollas highlighted, that offers new forms of creativity. This takes us further into the intersubjective and relational encounter of therapy that happens at a conscious, and more profoundly, an unconscious level. It is a call to go forth, paradoxically knowing and not-knowing, into a space of infinite complexity and sophistication.

Summary

Building on traditional understandings of the unconscious (Chapter 5), we saw important new developments in our awareness of the unconscious, including: the collective and mystical unconscious of Jung; the creative unconscious captured by Bollas, Benjamin, and Bion; the intersubjective and relational unconscious; the social unconscious of Foulkes; and the evolving unconscious that represents our encounter with the varieties of unconscious processes we work with as psychodynamic or integrative trainees or therapists. So what are the implicit beliefs dynamic therapists have about the unconscious and how does this profoundly shape their work? This is the subject of the next chapter.

Reflective questions

Which understanding of the unconscious most appeals to you, and which is the most challenging?

Taking the most challenging, what is it that we are resisting, consciously (which may reflect an unconscious process at work)?

How do you see aspects of the unconscious at work in clinical practice?

Looking at research

Meek, H. (2003) The place of the unconscious in qualitative research, *Forum Qualitative Sozialforschung/Forum: Qualitative Social Research*, 4(2). Available at: http://www.qualitative-research.net/index.php/fqs/article/view/711/1540

7

The implicit unconscious

In this chapter, we will examine the implicit beliefs that psychodynamic and integrative therapists have about the unconscious. As these are 'implicit', they are rarely, if ever, examined. Such beliefs, or unspoken assumptions, originate in our life stories but are often highlighted through our experience of professional training and personal therapy. We therefore soak them in without conscious realisation but act them out without having realised we believe them.

Annie's story

Annie was a client I saw for four years several times a week. Her history of extensive abuse from a very early age by her father and brother left her 'voiceless' – she couldn't assert herself and initially came to therapy in order to become more assertive with her male boss at work. I explained I didn't offer the kind of therapy that focused on solutions but that I wanted to hear her story and help her make sense of her life. This is a common approach for psychodynamic therapies, allowing the knowledge of the past to emerge in detail, with all its uncomfortable thoughts and feelings, and not simply the rehearsed story of our past. Unconscious thoughts and feelings emerge into consciousness through the relationship with the therapist expressed through transference and counter-transference (see Chapter 13).

Later, Annie said that, at some deep level, she felt safe as she sensed somehow that my story, even though this was not known to her, echoed some deep level of her own. She also went on to train as a psychodynamic therapist after I had moved away from the area.

A decade later, we bumped into one another at a residential conference. We sat one evening in the bar where, in a reflective mode, Annie said that she had learnt more about therapy from me than she had in her training course.

Annie's account of my therapy could be interpreted in many ways: a positive transference; a form of idealisation; an expression of splitting where I was the 'good breast' (something we will discuss later); or more likely, as I would see it now, an intersubjective encounter where something unique was created, an analytic third (we shall also explore this later). Our therapeutic encounter was a meeting of our unconsciousnesses, where my unconscious knew the contours and abyss of her unconscious and was willing to enter into a place of knowing, revealing, not-knowing, and containing that enabled Annie to feel a greater sense of wholeness.

What Annie illustrates and what unites new iterations of psychoanalysis, all forms of psychoanalytic psychotherapy, psychodynamic counselling, integrative approaches, and contemporary psychodynamic therapy is a belief in, and use of, conscious and unconscious processes. It is like an idea that transfixes our mind. It can be a tantalising glimpse etched in our memory of something 'other' and the unexpected emotions this brings. Every dynamic therapist has acquired a number of implicit beliefs about the unconscious, how they work with it, or it with them. This belief-making process has been through personal experience, sitting in a room or lying on a couch with their therapist, reading literature of all sorts, not just that required by the training course or therapeutic training itself, and last but certainly not least, learning from their clients. It is much clearer for everyone concerned to discover what these implicit beliefs about the unconscious might be and to make them explicit.

We might express this by way of an analogy. As a child, in a moment of enthusiasm, I decided to dismantle a watch that was not working. This, I discovered, was remarkably easy to achieve. However, confronted by a small bundle of cogs, I tried (unsuccessfully) to tension the spring to put it back where it had come from. This enterprise was doomed to failure. Later, when working in a psychiatric hospital, I saw how easy it was to pull apart another person's psyche, even with good intent. but, like the spring, the dismantled pieces remained for all to see, some broken beyond repair. Diving into the unconscious of another is not without risk and requires caution, a task that can be best done with proper preparation. Yet it is an engagement with the unconscious that is a unique part of the dancing landscape found in contemporary psychodynamic therapy and one with which all therapists in this field and the field of integrative therapy must engage.

Six core beliefs and practices

There are six simple but profound beliefs and practices psychodynamic therapists hold about, and perform in relation to, the unconscious and its use in their work. These vary in degree and according to circumstances but they are still present in our therapeutic work.

Belief One. Every person possesses an unconscious mental life or inner world that is part known and part unknown. This is the world of the mind, with its musings, memories, thinking, feeling, and dreaming, all paradoxically profound and bizarre at the same time. The unconscious aspect of us is constantly active and deeply influences all thinking and behaviour. Like a golden thread, the unconscious glitters with possibility in every person and every interaction. Yet it is also a tangle of conflicts, desires, fears, hopes, and dreams that we find difficult to acknowledge.

Kat's story

Kat was sent to me as a last resort. Such a referral always fills me with trepidation, as I cannot rescue people or become their emotional saviour. Kat was a 16-year-old with a complex history of eating issues, self-harm, and impulsive behaviours. Our work in the first six months was to get Kat to trust me, nothing more complex than that. I was never quite sure she would come back each week, as I sensed she was always ready to flee.

An unbidden thought came early on: 'What has so frightened you, you want to run and never stop?' This did not come from the work we were doing at that stage but I sensed it was what Kat was experiencing unconsciously, so I said it out loud. Kat felt that a part of her she did not really know or understand was being discovered in therapy. Kat would tell me things that were going on in her day-to-day life, and I would make interpretations connecting her external world with her internal world. Despite my never being sure she would turn up from week to week, she never missed a session. One day Kat told me she liked coming, as it helped her make sense of all what was going on.

Then she said, 'And I had this really cool dream, do you want to hear it?'

Often clients feel like they need to be given permission to explore this inner world. They regard the clinical setting as a warrant to explore their deepest and, potentially, darkest drives. It is also vital to underline that there are always two people, each with their own unconscious, in the room – both need expression, both need each other, both enter into forms of eurythmic movement. We dance with the unconscious and this is the art of all dynamically informed therapies. In our counselling room, there is a physical space created that allows for a psychic space in which it is safe to experiment, make mistakes, step on toes, and move in time and rhythm with each other. Some steps will be choreographed by the therapist's theoretical understanding (for example, by using directed questions arising from the clinical encounter to lead the client deeper into their past or unconscious), some will be spontaneous as the unconscious of two people emerge and interact, with recaptured memory and desire, old wounds and new healings, ghostly presences and transformed objects (for example, in free and unanticipated discussions and digressions). Regardless, both therapist and client should be touched at profound levels.

Belief Two. Psychodynamic therapies are intentional. The desire of every dynamic therapist is to bring about insight, understanding, or meaning so the client can be freed from previous unhelpful or maladaptive patterns. The client can choose how to proceed with authentic freedom, even if they choose to repeat something they did before, this time knowingly. This involves engaging with the unconscious to understand its yet-to-be revealed contents and to illuminate its opaque structures as experienced by that person. Each 'self' is a one-off designer piece, and psychodynamic therapists bring to this work their own 'self', including their unconscious processes. We do not stumble across the unconscious by blind accident; we do need to be in the vicinity.

Let's consider another analogy. Joe Cornish is a British landscape photographer who has taken some wonderful pictures of Scottish mountains (2009). Having climbed many of the same peaks, I realise that he must have camped on or near the summit overnight so as to be in the right place at the right time to get his desired image. Similarly, psychodynamic therapists intend to encounter their desired object, the unconscious – elusive though this can be – and this requires them to have prepared to be in the right place at the right time, to even allow the potential 'picture' that has been shaped in their mind to be encountered (or not encountered, as the case may be) in reality.

Belief Three. The multifaceted work of a psychodynamic therapist is elusive but can be captured metaphorically. We capture the 'feel' of this process through a range of metaphors linked to other roles or professions. The metaphors we choose or integrate, however, might also tell us something about our unconscious associations concerning how each of us inhabits the role of being a psychodynamic therapist. No one metaphor is better than another.

We work variously as:

- an archaeologist – excavating the past held in the unconscious;
- a detective – solving mysteries based on the clues yet to be linked to identify the causes or culprits;
- a priest – offering a safe place for darker aspects to be revealed, like a confessional without absolution;
- a mountain guide – traversing the ridges and peaks of a psychological landscape, helping people by relying on their experience and expertise, especially when the cloud descends;
- an architect – building something creative that blends the past with the future;
- a picture restorer – stripping away the accretions of years of grime to reveal what lies beneath, restoring the object (or person) to its original colours and patching torn or frayed canvas;
- a dancing partner – learning with a new partner how they will find innovative steps and interpretations of classical behaviours; and
- a poet – working with words, images, or symbols in their pared down elemental form to resonate with others.

Contemporary psychodynamic therapy gets below the surface to reveal what is hidden, but the experience of doing this offers surprises, and a form of aliveness, for the therapist and client alike. Psychodynamic therapists also work as interpreters, not of foreign language, but of the unconscious. They do this through using glimpses of the unconscious revealed through dreams, slips of the tongue, 'forgetting', transference (an unconscious process where a client sees another person as if they are a significant person from their past), counter-transference (drawing on the therapist's experience of, and reaction to, the patient, consciously and unconsciously), and a similar but unique process of 'projective identification' (see Chapter 14). A psychodynamic therapist works with the words, images, and feelings taken from the conscious and unconscious worlds of the client to find a language that speaks to that person's inner and outer worlds with shared meaning. In a dancing landscape model, no one of these analogous professions is the 'right' one, although all require uncommon skill.

Belief Four. Contemporary psychodynamic therapy holds to the tradition that a personal experience of therapy is an indispensable element of preparation for the therapist role. It is important to offer reasons why this is the case rather than 'we've always done it that way'. It is one 'implicit' belief that is rarely questioned.

One key reason is that, historically, psychoanalysis, psychoanalytic psychotherapy, and analytical psychology have worked on the basis of an apprenticeship model – that we learn how to be a therapist by receiving therapy, whether we think we need it or not. (This tradition is also found in counselling psychology and integrative, humanistic, and dynamic therapies.). This is the primary reason why most cognitive-trained therapists do not need to have therapy as part of their training. They are not suffering from depression, anxiety, OCD, eating disorders, or the other health conditions and symptoms they treat. They are working from a medical model of human nature, viewing the world in terms of diagnosis and treatment; they assess what would be effective for the client based on their needs at a given moment (Roth and Fonagy 2005). Where they are less effective is when a person wants to make sense of an event, their past, and how they live now.

Kat (who we saw earlier) had seen several cognitive therapists before me through Child and Adolescent Mental Health Services (CAMS) who aimed at reducing her self-harm and impulsive behaviours. I am not suggesting that my work with her was better than that with others, as she still had many challenging issues including feeling suicidal, but she did now have a sense of who she was, a person rather than a problem. How does my experience of therapy help a client like Kat? I recall taking a long time to trust my first therapist, well over twelve months. He waited patiently and the gentle but firm holding of me found an echo in what I was able to do with Kat. The issue was not to fix her problems, but to attend to her psyche, as mine had once been attended to. I knew the terrain and my hope is that is sufficient for now. Intriguingly, I still think about her, but sometimes with a deep concern.

In February 2014, while climbing alone and descending the north face of Tryfan, I slipped and fell 150 feet (Ross 2014) resulting in seven fractures to legs, ankles, and wrist plus a head injury, hypothermia, torn knee cartilages, and multiple cracked/bruised ribs; I spent some weeks in hospital. When seeing the consultant orthopaedic surgeon, who was doing a final check on me before discharge, he asked what I did as a job. When I replied, 'Professor of Psychotherapy at Oxford University', he said 'I don't know what a psychotherapist is'. I talked about trauma related to accidents and their psychological effect. He looked shocked and said, 'Surely, once the helicopter had rescued you and taken you to the hospital all your trauma was over'. One reviewer wrote on my draft text that this comment didn't ring true as it was 'implausibly naive'. Unfortunately, it was verbatim. This surgeon viewed the world in a very distinct way and, deciding he had reached the limit of his empathy, turned to his computer screen and said, 'Now, looking at your x-rays . . .'. He was back on safe ground, away from these messy feelings and emotions, yet if we hold to the vital importance of the unconscious, we are unconscious of the reasons why we need therapy that will only be revealed if we have that therapy. After my accident, I did go back into therapy as this present-day trauma, and my responses to it, uncovered very early-embodied feelings related to a similarly life-threatening event in my premature birth. I needed someone who would look at the hidden past and connect it to my present, not simply declare me fit because I could stand unaided on formerly broken legs and ankles. Another deeper, long-distant part of me was fractured, residing in the unconscious, waiting for discovery. I still try and climb mountains, albeit more slowly and with less strength and flexibility in my ankles, but these days always go with another person and often a guide. A local guide knows the rock, the routes, the micro-climate weather systems, the dangers, and offers safety in that knowledge. They have been there before many times. They also offer companionship. I can still recall one guide, a normally taciturn Scotsman, put his arm around my shoulder and say, 'It's so good to see a father with his son' as my son, Toby, and I completed the Cullins on Skye. The therapist, when external to the cognitive- and medically-based approaches, is just such a wise guide. We can know about the contours of another's unconscious because we have explored our own. We know that our unconscious is not the same as that of our clients, but we have a sense of how the land lies. The same dynamic processes will have been at work. We have encountered our own subterfuges, defences, denials, actings out, enactments, avoidance of the dread experience of the abyss, and falling into regression fearing we would never recover.

Many training courses have personal therapy as an essential requirement for this reason. Yet this raises the thorny question of, 'Do you really benefit from therapy if you are required to do so?' (Jacobs 2011). While it is always more helpful to choose something for oneself, as it brings an emotional commitment to the task, the answer is 'yes'. A student on a psychotherapy training course came to me for therapy because it was a requirement of her course. In a moment of honesty, she admitted that deep down she always knew she needed and wanted therapy but somehow couldn't give herself permission to undergo it. However, by going on a course that required this, she was able to overcome that obstacle. Needless to say, we did work on this issue in the therapy.

This raises another related question, 'How often should I be in therapy?' The frequency is often set by different dynamic trainings, although some clients choose to stay longer based on what they discover of their internal world. Unlike psychoanalysis, however, contemporary psychodynamic therapy does not view the frequency of therapy as inviolable, a supposedly heretical idea first adopted by Lacan. While Freud advocated psychoanalysis as an intensive process of up to six sessions a week, the time period may have only lasted months rather than years.

So, while there are variations in the frequency and length of time in therapy, what unites all therapy is the presence and power of the unconscious. Every form of therapy I have been through (ranging from once a month to three times a week) has involved discovering more about, and being receptive to, unconscious processes. Each has been helpful in their distinctive ways and was what I needed at that time, although discovering aspects that we have repressed are not pain-free encounters.

Belief Five. It may sound paradoxical given Belief Four; nevertheless, we need to be able to believe in the unconscious – but not too much. A belief in the unconscious is a conviction based on evidence, evidence that some dispute. I cannot categorically offer proof of the existence of the unconscious in a reductive scientific form. Yet, psychoanalysis and the unconscious can be believed in as both philosophically and scientifically valid (Lacewing 2013). The opposite extreme would be to attribute almost everything as springing from the unconscious. While this is unlikely, I have observed an over-attribution to the unconscious that borders on the unbelievable. There are dangers in viewing everything as driven and dominated by the unconscious, as it robs us of agency and humanity. As Phillips claimed, psychoanalysis and the unconscious, if viewed as a fundamental religion, is 'notably insufficient' (1994: 138). Dynamic therapies and their underlying theories require faith, but not blind obedience, a denial of reality, or an over-attribution of the theories to the experiences we have in the clinical setting. We need to believe in the unconscious so that the voices of the past can be heard, but not so reify that past that we only hear these voices, ignoring the significant chatter of ordinary and everyday life.

Belief Six. There is always something to be discovered, which requires occupying an epistemic space of knowing and not-knowing. Joan Riviere, one of the earliest women analysts in Britain and a translator of Freud, recounts a fragment of her short analysis with Freud:

It is as necessary to keep in mind how strong the not seeing and not knowing is in us to learn all we can about what is unconscious in the mind . . . In my analysis he one day made some interpretation, and I responded to it by an objection. He then said: 'it is un-conscious.' I was overwhelmed then by the realisation that I knew nothing about it . . . in that instant he had created in me his discovery of the powerful unconscious in our minds that we know nothing of, and that yet is impelling and directing us.

(quoted in Sutherland 1989: 148f.)

Yet not-knowing something can be difficult. A client can so intrigue us with their story that we want to know more. Like a psychodynamic soap-opera, we end each week's episode on a cliff-hanger with a passing remark made in the last five minutes or even as the client has their hand on the door-handle ready to leave the room. So the following week our curiosity is aroused, our psyche expectant, and we are tempted to start 'So how did you get on . . .' rather than sit in silence, waiting, offering space, neither uninterested nor intruding. Bion believed we should enter each therapeutic session without memory, desire, or understanding, making every session unique without a past history or a future plan, in order to let unconscious intuition be at work (Bion 1970). What was Bion thinking when he said those words that at first glance seem rather strange? Memories are about the past, desires are about the future, understanding is about the mind, but psychodynamic work is in the encounter of the present, conscious, and unconscious, where we become attuned to the unconscious expressed through what Bion called 'acts of faith'. He defined this as:

[the therapist's ability or capacity (a skill that is still in the process of development) to have faith in] certain ideas, hunches or intuitions that suddenly emerge in the therapeutic space. It implies the capacity to accept the absolute truth, the existence of O as an ultimate reality, in order to structure an interpretation. Being able to reach such an attitude will depend on the analyst's discipline of listening while avoiding using any memory or desire.

(López-Corvo 2003: 22)

Out of this experience of not-knowing, by waiting we give space for an unexpected intuition that in that moment illuminates the work and makes it come alive. Consequently, not-knowing is a crucial feature of psychodynamic therapists' engagement with the unconscious.

These six implicit beliefs about the unconscious are made explicit to aid the work of all psychodynamic therapists. It makes anyone working this way, exclusively or integratively, attentive to the unconscious in unique ways (see Table 7.1).

A vital part of psychodynamic working is to be able to hold the other person in mind. This does not mean you are consciously thinking about them all the time but, in essence, through the unconscious, we are. Each client has the potential to be part of us and to make us more than we were before. They are our engagement with what or whom Levinas calls the 'Other' (Orange 2010). Yet we need models, ways of thinking to help us do this. We are engaging with multiple models that move in and out through dynamic entanglements, or as I imagine it the dancing landscape of the unconscious, full of chaos and complexity out of which comes newly discovered or re-discovered life. Our clients come with their own unconscious and it may not fit with the unconscious we have in mind. For example, whilst traditionally most self-identifying Freudians would reject Jung's collective and mythological unconscious because it did not fit Freud's model of the mind, many people do believe in it. It makes sense to them and forms a way they experience life. If we 'close down' our ability to even acknowledge this as a possibility, we do them a disservice and diminish our opportunity to enter into new encounters with the unconscious.

Table 7.1 The implicit beliefs of psychodynamic therapy

Belief One: Every person possesses an unconscious mental life or inner world that is part known and part unknown.

Belief Two: Psychodynamic therapies are intentional.

Belief Three: The multifaceted work of a psychodynamic therapist is elusive, but can be captured metaphorically.

Belief Four: Contemporary psychodynamic therapy holds to the tradition that a personal experience of therapy is an indispensable element of preparation for the role of therapist.

Belief Five: We need to be able to believe in the unconscious – but not too much.

Belief Six: There is always something to be discovered, which requires occupying an epistemic space of knowing and not-knowing.

Summary

A key challenge old and new therapists face is to understand the unconscious and name our implicit beliefs about it. We need to see how these implicit beliefs or ideas shape our practice. This allows us as psychodynamic therapists to be ready to be in the room with the client, consciously and unconsciously. But who exactly is it that faces us in the therapeutic space between the two chairs? Who are they, and more importantly, how did they become who they are? We need to explore how human beings develop from life in the womb, through birth, and into the early months and years of infant development. This follows the psychoanalytic tradition of linking psychological development and physical development, as this forms the cradle from which we emerge as a person, become a self, and learn to possess our unique mind–body unity, which the next chapter will explore.

Reflective questions

Thinking about your own therapy or work with clients, or accounts that you have studied, which of these six aspects (Belief Three) of the unconscious have you encountered?

Knowing about these six implicit beliefs, how can you make them more explicit in your current or future work?

From your experience, are there other forms of the unconscious that you have identified as implicit in your thinking or practice?

Looking at research

We have implicit biases about many things. Whilst I have focused on the unconscious, there is an online research project on implicit bias in which you can participate. Available at: https://implicit.harvard.edu/implicit/research/ [accessed 10 October 2018].

PART 3
How We Develop

8

The infant unconscious – Oedipus, bad breasts, lines, and stages

Having made the exciting discovery that there is an aspect within us that is both conscious and unconscious, how does this shape the way we develop as human beings? Where does Josh get his imagination from when he tells me about monsters under his bed, some that are friendly, but others that are fierce? Why does 24-month-old Adil never sleep for more than four hours a night? What can Alix do about her past? Her mother committed suicide when she was aged two and all she has are shadowy memories. As an adult, she fears she too will be depressed like her mother and do something calamitous, but she doesn't know what. How is it that these individuals become the people they are, and are in the process of becoming? Are they trapped in a past, like unwelcome guests in a dark, abandoned mansion so loved by horror movies, waiting for something bad to happen? Has a person's past, mysterious and forgotten, lost in the mists of childhood, established the foundations of the person they are today? How can we be so influenced by events and relationships occurring before we possess language and therefore are unable to ascribe any meaning in words? How much of this is the experience of just being a baby, or a child, engaged in the ordinary process of development? What else might be going on in their minds?

Answers to these profound and personal questions can be found in a psychodynamic understanding of human development and one of the unique ideas found in psychoanalysis – the past influences the present. The more we know about the past, the greater insight this can give to understanding the person sitting in front of us.

Patterns from the past

When discussing creativity and imagination, Freud (1908) noted we use patterns from the past, in the present, to construct a future. Some of these patterns were set even before birth (Piontelli 1992). While these templates are not deterministic, they do offer a pattern for our thinking and feelings, which become active when we encounter a new experience or find ourselves in a new situation. Every day we are involved in a dynamic process of balancing the past, the present, and the future in working out who we are, what we are doing, and why.

Zoe's story

As a child, Zoe was a lone girl in the car, with her father doing his rounds as a GP in a rural county. Now as an adult she is anxious but doesn't know why.

Forty years later, Zoe returns to Northumbria and, on a hot summer's day, is sitting in the car. She suddenly becomes overwhelmed by powerful feelings of anger, being scared like a child, and feeling pain in different parts of her body. This was the trigger for Zoe to enter therapy – something she had thought about doing for a long time but had always been held back by a nagging thought, 'Mustn't tell'.

Zoe's crushing anxieties were signposts pointing to something traumatic that had happened in her inner world, with the embodied nature of trauma linking this to a pre-verbal stage of development. Some things are so painful, the unconscious protects us by excluding them from consciousness.

What emerged through the interactions in the relationship (interactions including transference, counter-transference, and projective identification, as well as other forms of enactment) established that she had been subject to early childhood sexual abuse by her father from around the age of three until she was eleven when she went to boarding school. At school, Zoe was bullied and she was angry with her mother for sending her away, as she had been the driving force in making Zoe leave home. Now she understood her mother had been trying to protect her. Therapy helped Zoe to realise her anger at her mother also related to the fact that she must have 'known' about the abuse but did nothing to stop it. Her sense of loss at being sent to boarding school was not just because she was bullied but also because she loved and hated her father. In the therapy, Zoe expressed a great deal of confusion, not knowing what was true or untrue, as well as many conflicted feelings including her need to hold in her molten rage. Zoe's early experiences have had a profound influence on her life. The past still haunts her and her fear is that she is like a buried landmine waiting to be triggered, exploding, maiming anyone too close. For Zoe, the trigger was waiting in a car on a hot summer's day in an 'old' location that released destructive memories, one aftershock after another. While she could physically drive home, she did so mechanically, overwhelmed by vivid memories beginning to surface. For Zoe, the past is all too present.

The unconscious in and beyond the womb

We can understand Zoe's story, but there are parts of our own story and the stories of others that go further back than childhood, to birth itself, and, as we will see, prior even to life in the womb (Raphael-Leff 2015). Understanding birth is complicated enough but our story doesn't begin at birth. When does that unique sense of self, expressed as consciousness, and by inference, the unconscious, begin? Twin research can help us. Piontelli's (1992) unique research used ultrasound technology to record the movements and interactions of three singletons and four sets of twins in the womb, followed by observational studies up to the age of four, with further brief observations up to the age of six. Although ultrasounds cannot tell us what a foetus feels or thinks, the movements suggest some form of self–other identity activation coming from a sense of an inner world. This continued as Piontelli observed that forms of connection and movement in twins in utero were also played out after birth in the early years. Observations from the ages of four to six show a change, with the earlier experience of the womb becoming a rich source of phantasy, supporting Klein's (1923) perception of the importance of this aspect of early development (Likierman 2002).

Woodward's (1998) work on lone twins is similarly pioneering. In her training as a psychoanalytic psychotherapist, none of her analysts or therapists took seriously the loss of her identical twin when she was aged three. Driven to understand this experience, she initiated a research project in which over 200 lone twins were interviewed (known as 'twinless twins' in the USA, or twins whose counterpart dies in utero or at the point of birth). Woodward discovered that lone twins carry an on-going, unexplained, and barely expressible loss even if their twin died in utero or at birth. Lone twins sense an identity existing in the womb, a finding supported by Hayton (2007). These accounts support the idea of a conscious and unconscious self that exists before birth.

For some, the origins of the psyche go far back in time to many generations before birth. How we relate and the patterns we experience run through families, their ability to function or perpetuate dysfunction, family traditions, disintegrations, migrations, and feuds. These form a psychological backdrop for the expectant mother, carrying her child, physically and emotionally, in the womb. As Rucker and Mermelstein observe:

> The creation of a child's psyche is begun many generations before his birth. The patterns of relating that evolve in his early relationship with his mother have their roots in the relationships of his ancestors, and he becomes heir to the family traditions. Even before his birth his personality is partly moulded, because the personalities of his parents are existing entities. He is born into a family with specific needs and structure, and he is nurtured before and after birth by a mother who has a specific psychological constellation. The innumerable potentialities for character development, which are inherent in every human being, are thus naturally and necessarily limited and refined by a process that begins long before conception.
>
> (1979: 147)

Understanding the past to help in the present

In a psychodynamic approach, the more we can know and understand about the past, the more we can help in the present. When asked, clients often say they cannot remember anything about their childhood or that they had a wonderful childhood. With the right encouragement, memories – both good and bad – emerge as clients re-visit their past and describe their truth.

Tess's story

I started to work with Tess after an attempted suicide. Her doctor put her on antidepressants, but also suggested a 'talking therapy' and referred her to me. Tess had read up about therapy and wanted to do the 'kind of therapy that looks at the past' before going on to say, 'I had a very happy childhood'.

Each week, Tess filled in a self-report form rating the level of her depression (PHQ-9 – see Zoe's story in Chapter 3 for more on this). I asked her how she found this. Tess said that it was the one part of her week when she stopped her hectic round of manic activity making the most of student life. The form was helpful as it made her realise she was depressed and there were times when she 'crashed', the last time being the suicide attempt. However, as her story unfolded, Tess realised that, while there were times when she was happy, there were dark holes she avoided.

What emerged was an unresolved grief at the loss of her grandmother at the time when her parents were divorcing. Tess recalled, 'She always had time for me and wanted to know about my world. I could tell her anything. I felt safe there'. Tess cried, racking sobs filled the room, and a buried emotional past was dug up as a present and painful reality.

Something had happened in Tess's psychological development that left her troubled. The earliest understandings of the self were viewed as the person's mind encompassing the whole person, which emerged from psychoanalysts working with adults and thinking back to the early experience of an infant. Psychoanalysis is a science of observation and interpretation in the living experiment of the consulting room with willing research participants (Lacewing 2013). It is, therefore, as we saw in Chapter 3, a field with a nuanced evidence base combining quantitative and qualitative inputs. Such case-study observations have validity but need to be held in tandem with newly emerging ideas based on infant observation and neuroscientific insights, which have the benefits of testability, repeatability, and reliability, although the interpretation of some neuroscientific findings on human development is complex and not always very accessible.

Yet the paradox remains that these new insights alone are not sufficient to help re-create, repair, or engage with what clients seek in dynamic therapies. The past is still to be encountered – it has been waiting patiently for a long time. The infant cries are not distant echoes but, growing in volume, they need to be heard; the hungry ghosts need to become welcomed and invited to become valued ancestors; the undead of the psyche need to be released for a proper burial. In short, our internal working models need to be identified and, if necessary, modified.

Psychodynamic thinking evolved a developmental theory about how and why we become the people we are. Starting with Freud's Oedipal ideas, these have been adapted by such later analytic thinkers as Klein, Erikson, Winnicott, and Mahler. Arising out of psychoanalytic thinking, but distinct from it, Bowlby (along with Ainsworth and Main) developed attachment theory. Further advances in infant observation and developmental psychology led to Stern's interpersonal theories (the development of the self through multiple self-states), and have been continued by Tronick (1989, 2007), Beebe (2014; Beebe and Lachmann 2014), and the Boston Change Process Study Group (BCPSG 2010). These later developments are supported by the findings of developmental neuroscience (Kenny 2013), made accessible by Gerhardt (2015).

We will begin with Freud before turning to Erikson. The following chapter will examine Bowlby, Stern, and the BCPSG. First, however, let us discuss the nature of babies.

The nature of babies

What is it like to be a baby?

We have all been a baby, so at one level we know. We also, of course, don't know and cannot recall. As adults, we cannot shrink back into our bodies or poke around the inside of our brains in order to recall our thinking and feeling. While there are some humanistic therapies that focus on regression, re-birthing, and primal integration (Rowan and Dryden 1988), the way most of us sense how we once were comes in one of two ways. The first is through photographs and stories. The mysterious art of great photography is to reveal more than what appears on the surface. The image resonates with us and, as we look at pictures of our childhood, we can sense something 'other', often being transported back in time, across places and emotions. I look at the earliest pictures of me as a baby and I experience 'help-lessness'. I see another image of me standing up against a tree and have a memory of learning to walk aged about twelve months, but is this possible? While it is commonly accepted that children have few accessible memories before the age of three, such research is based on asking the question, 'What is your earliest memory?' If an artefact is present, such as a photograph, even earlier memories are elicited, although photographs often include the family story associated with it (e.g. 'We took that picture when you were one, learning to walk'). So my memory is in fact a construction of several factors but I have a feeling or sense of that experience different from the account.

Megan's story

Megan, a client who had a history of terrifying sexual abuse perpetrated by her father, once asked if I could 'hold' a picture for her. It was the one and only picture she had of herself. Her father discovered she loved playing with the tin box containing the family photographs and looking at pictures of herself as a child. Megan recalls he found her playing, calmly took the tin from her, took out the pictures of her and burnt them one by one in front of her. That was apart from the very one I was holding, the one photograph she was able to hide. This picture represented a time when she was happy, despite the psychological carnage of the family. While she was still being abused at this age, she felt it was minor compared to the later abuse.

Several years later, Megan, who was moving away and starting a new relationship, asked if she could have her photograph back as she felt she could now hold it safely herself. While photographs can serve as an emotional snapshot of our past, much of our past is unknown, so what emerges comes from some intuitive part of a self-experience shaped by our personal encounters.

Re-discovering being a baby

The second way we re-discover what it is to be a baby is by having our own child (or children) or seeing babies in a family, social, or professional context. They trigger unexpected emotions we find difficult to put into words, so psychodynamic theorists from Freud onwards put these experiences into conceptual ideas. In trying to reconstruct the world of the infant, they could only use themselves or their patients. Their thinking reflects both originality and, at times, psychopathology. Every developmental theory comes from a theorist who is searching for their all too elusive self, and some also become therapists.

Freud's theories

Developmental theory

Freud originated a developmental theory that balanced the function of the mind, the psychological drives it contains, alongside the physical development of the body. The adult patients he saw in his consulting room influenced Freud's thinking. Most of them were female, had distressing physical symptoms, but could recall traumatic childhoods, often involving sexual exploitation. His understanding of their psychopathology took him back to the origins of the psychological processes that accounted for their disturbing symptoms. He theorised about how we can experience something that leads to both normal and pathological development. Pathology occurs when a crucial psychological stage is not fully negotiated in childhood.

Freud's ideas, expressed in summary form, are often caricatures or distortions of his thinking. His ideas are rarely simple and, in trying to reduce them in order to make them accessible, this potentially robs the reader of encountering their complexity, richness, and originality of thought. While it is best to read original Freud, this too has its challenges, as Freud was writing over a hundred years ago and his writing reflects his time. Why are these ideas important? They underline the reality that we live and act at conscious and unconscious levels all the time. There is a constant dynamic interplay, and this disturbs us. We are swayed by impulses and desires that make no rational sense; we avoid areas of life that trigger powerful, unwanted feelings; we fear we are always one short step away from disintegration. Many of our clients come with lives haunted by past events. While these events may have been traumatic, it is the nature of the haunting that is disturbing. The ghosts of the psyche are hungry ghosts that compulsively repeat toxic relationships or problematic thoughts and actions and become locked in the past, imprisoned with feelings that will not go away, or locked in the present unable to connect with all that has gone before. For Freud, the solution was to see how his theories translated into how we develop as a person – biologically, socially, and psychologically – in the context of the family or care context of our origin.

Sexuality

Freud's developmental theory is built on his understanding of sexuality, which is much broader than the evolutionary drives for mating and survival of the species. He viewed sexuality as the formative way human beings develop and express themselves, involving the body and the mind, present from birth. His view of infantile sexuality (Freud 1905a) was considered scandalous because, until then, sexuality was considered an adult experience with a focus on the genitals and the primacy of sexual intercourse. Freud's view of infantile sexuality was that children know no constraint in seeking pleasure and find this in every part of their body. He called infants 'polymorphously perverse' and, despite its negative connotations today, Freud meant their desire for satisfaction was fluid, interchangeable, moving from one source or area to another as required. Infants experience 'the most intense pleasure, disappointment, and pain. The skin, smell, gaze, the act of suckling, or even excreting, and body warmth can yield a dividend of psychic enjoyment' (Pick 2015: 37). While we could add spitting, biting, and touching to this list, this cluster of phenomena points to the importance of primary eroticism through skin-to-skin contact experienced by the infant with the mother. (I use the term 'mother' to refer to a person with a generic, inclusive non-binary meaning.) The role of the 'mother' is to offer physical and psychological well-being for the dependent infant to survive, then thrive. The quality of this relationship, and the powerful feelings it evokes, is especially formative.

Initially the mouth, then later the anus and genitals offer particular sources of pleasure for an infant as they contain a concentration of nerve endings (also found in other parts of the body, termed 'erogenous zones'). A baby commonly puts everything in its mouth as a way of discovering information, working out if it is pleasurable. For example, trying to feed a baby sprouts (adult rationalisation – green, healthful, source of vitamins C and K) gets the common response of them being spat out, with an accompanying scrunched up face that says non-verbally, 'Why did you do that to me? How could you be so cruel?' The oral, anal, and genital stages mark infant development through to early childhood. Metaphorically, these represent what a child can gain control of, and use, as a means of expressing who they are.

Emmy's story

Emmy was a three-year-old who had been in foster care but was now being adopted. Her birth mother was a drug addict and suffered with sustained mental health issues. It was suspected not only that Emmy had been neglected but also she may have been abused by one of her mother's many 'friends'.

Emmy would compulsively masturbate, obviously meeting an emotional need and finding comfort in the physical sensations of her body. As a child, she was extremely needy and required specialist help from a child psychotherapist to start to address her issues. Her compulsive and inappropriate masturbation stopped when she realised that the people around her were not going to leave her, although clearly there would be many challenges to face around attachment.

Introducing Oedipus

Jacobs (1986, 2012) views Freud's psycho-sexual stages through the psychological patterns that are being played out based on early childhood experiences. The oral stage becomes the theatre of trust and dependency; the anal stage highlights authority and control; and the genital stage hosts the drama of sexuality and rivalry played out in the Oedipus complex understood mythically and symbolically (Jacobs 1986). Jacobs re-configured these as: trust and attachment; authority and autonomy; and co-operation and competition, respectively (Jacobs 2012).

While Freud's psycho-sexual stages seem rather contrived, they were revolutionary at their time in linking the external world with the evolution of the person's internal world. Freud, having built the stages for the development of a person, brings them all together, like

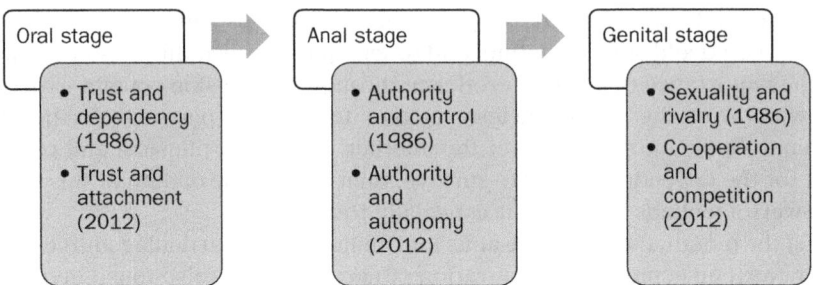

Figure 8.1 Freud's psycho-sexual stages in Jacobs

the Last Night of the Proms, in the climactic Oedipus complex that became the crown jewels of psychoanalytic theory.

The story of Oedipus is worth hearing. It is a universal story of tragedy, truth, and what we are blind to. In summary, the story of the Oedipus begins with tragedy and ends in tragedy, only this time round Oedipus knows the truth. His parents were warned that their son was destined to murder his own father. After being maimed by a spike, Oedipus is left to die, only to be rescued by a shepherd, then later adopted by monarchs. Oedipus believes the latter to be his parents but, when this is questioned, he consults an oracle. Oedipus is told he will kill his father and marry his mother. Oedipus flees to protect his 'adoptive' parents but, in his travels, he quarrels with and accidently kills a stranger who, unbeknown to Oedipus, is his father, Laius. Oedipus later solves riddles posed by a Sphinx that result in him being rewarded by being made King, marrying Jocasta, his mother. With his father murdered and his mother his wife, a plague descends on the city. Oedipus agrees to find the murderer, but when he finds the blood on his hands, he blinds himself and Jocasta, his mother, commits suicide. Oedipus is led away by his children into metaphorical darkness. Bettelheim adds Oedipus,

> was unaware of his innermost feelings . . . [We encounter the idea that] having one's sight turned away from [the] external world and directed inwards – toward the inner nature of things – gives true knowledge and permits understanding of what is hidden and needs to be known.

> (1982: 23f.)

Oedipus and beyond

Freud found in Sophocles' *Oedipus Rex* a dramatic play of universal significance that touched his own life and, by extension, the lives of others influenced by his own creation, psychoanalysis. For Freud, the story of the psyche was to prove every bit as dramatic. He wrote to his early friend and confidante, Wilhelm Fliess, in 1897:

> Everyone in the audience was once a budding Oedipus in fantasy and each recoils in horror from the dream fulfilment here translated into reality, with the full quality of repression which separated his infantile state from his present one.

> (Masson 1985: 272)

Freud believed that in the phallic phase of psycho-sexual development, a son desires his mother, wishing to possess her. Yet he is also afraid of the father who has the power to forbid him, which is experienced as 'castration anxiety'. The boy therefore represses his desire for the mother, undergoes a period of latency, before discovering it is safe to express his own desire for girls/women, not mothers, in adolescence. Freud believed he could account for the origins of gender and sexuality; instead, it reveals him as 'an early twentieth century slightly frustrated patriarchal white northern European male' (Barden 2015). While Freud was widely accepting of the breadth of sexuality for his time, the workings of the Oedipus complex privileges a male-dominated heterosexual perspective with little understanding of gay, lesbian, trans, or other non-aligned perspectives. So for most of the twentieth century, anyone wanting to train as an analyst either with a religious faith or a non-heterosexual orientation was considered as having insufficiently resolved their Oedipal conflicts.

Oedipus today

Contemporary attitudes to the Oedipus complex vary from: literal acceptance; an acceptance but also the recognition it needs to be adapted to work in practice; being understood as a powerful metaphor; to critical rejection as it denies the experience of many people. What it does do very powerfully, in a way that reflects the original play, is to remind us of the sheer force and power of feelings experienced by a child as they grow into a complex world they have never experienced before. This experience they take into adulthood. The Oedipus complex speaks to the lived experience of children. They are passionate, desiring, aggressive, irritating, obsessional, competitive, sexual (innocent enough unless abused), with the very parents on whom they rely. These states are experienced simultaneously, all wrapped up in one bundle like a baby in a big bath-towel. So, through the Oedipus complex, children learn about inclusion and exclusion, what is acceptable or permitted, and what is not. They form a psychological template about what fits with the society they are in, with its laws, rules, and regulations.

Britton (1998; Britton et al. 1989) made an important contribution that Oedipal thinking and experiencing enables a child to relate not just to another (two-person thinking) but *others* (three-person thinking) and this becomes an internal triangle in the mind that links the child and parents and influences all relating. This internal triangle also fosters the growth of knowledge, mental life, belief, and creativity.

Despite the wide disparity of views on the Oedipus complex, this concept illustrates the value of a dancing landscape model, which encourages entering into the theoretical space of the Oedipus complex, to inhabit it and to discover new paths, new adaptations that enrich the psychodynamic habitat (Britton et al. 1989; Verhaeghe 2009; Barden 2015; Fear 2015). The Oedipus complex is significant in terms of the dynamic experienced in the inner world, the vital importance of negotiating triangular relationships, and learning how we own and negotiate power. However, in its original formulation, it does not give a sufficiently accurate or nuanced account of the development of the person to be the sole means of psychodynamic understanding. For this, we need to turn to others, beginning with Klein.

Klein's love, hate, loss, and phantasy

The first person to adapt Freud's psycho-sexual stages was Melanie Klein. She focused on an earlier stage of development where her pre-Oedipal dynamics drew attention to the vital role of the mother, rather than simply the father, so dominant in Freud's thinking. This opened the way for the mother–baby constellation to become central to psychological and psychic development.

Klein's understanding of unconscious phantasy as a mental representation of something we experienced or needed enriched our thinking about what goes on in the mind (Hayman 1989). The clues to the origins of Klein's theories lay in the complexities of her own life. Discovering the writings of Freud led her to analysis with Ferenczi and the attention of Abraham. Abraham became a great supporter and his death in 1925 was an immense loss to her. He had started to develop ideas about how infants suck and gain satisfaction with a healthy sense of being, but also bite, leading to the removal of the breast and the sense of destruction of a partial love object. In loving and hating the object, ambivalence is introduced at a very early stage. Abraham combined drive theory with the emerging object relations approach and was the first to introduce the idea of the 'bad mother' (May 2001).

These ideas proved hugely significant for the development of Klein's theories. Klein's theory of the mind placed less emphasis on the biological stages advocated by Freud. Klein's infants construct a world in their mind: she called this 'phantasy', which is every bit as real as the external world. Klein placed the emergence of the Oedipus complex much earlier than Freud with the internal world full of destructive, murderous fantasies and images, often of death. 'For Freud, the child is a selfish savage; for Klein, it is a murderous cannibal' (Gay 1998: 468).

Carol's story

A friend of a friend, Carol, asked to see me as she knew I was a therapist and said she wanted some advice because she was concerned about her six-year-old daughter, Joy. Joy had been disruptive at school and had become obsessed with death, only wanting to wear black.

Joy had been referred to a child psychotherapist where Carol had sat in on the first assessment session. In the course of the assessment, it emerged that Joy was a twin whose fraternal twin brother had died in utero. After establishing a good relationship with Joy, the therapist said to her, 'Do you feel bad because you were a very hungry baby and you ate your brother?' Carol was shocked. Yet Joy was not, if anything she seemed relieved. It was as if somebody had reached deep into the world of her unconscious phantasy and spoken out loud what she was feeling but for which she lacked words. Such a seemingly stark interpretation had the effect of containing powerful and primitive feelings that existed in the mind. As the therapist contained Joy's phantasy, Joy learnt how to contain her own feelings, enabling her to settle into school.

Good and bad breasts

Klein's developmental model, rather than using phases or stages, adopted the idea of 'positions'. The whole of life revolves around oscillating between two positions. The paranoid-schizoid position comes with splitting, envy, good and bad breasts, and expelling unwanted sadistic and destructive feelings through projection. The depressive position is an acceptance that we will never acquire the object of our phantasy, where we can accept those close to us being a whole object metaphorically good and bad (hence the term 'depressive') yet live productively and creatively.

For Klein, the baby's mental world functions, at its most primitive level, in a phantasy that there are two mothers. These split between the 'good' – the mother that offers holding, warmth, touch, comfort, and being fed; and the 'bad' – the mother that is unavailable and unresponsive when the baby feels abandoned, as well as not giving the baby enough leaving her hungry, wet, or in discomfort. In the mind of the baby, they love the good mother, symbolised by the object of the 'good breast', and hate the bad mother, symbolised by the 'bad breast'. The baby wants to take in the good and expel the bad. Klein described this divided experience as the 'paranoid-schizoid position', the word paranoid conveying that this is a fantasy, a distortion of reality. Through this internal template, the baby engages with the external world, testing its reality. Here the powerful dynamics of the Oedipus story are at work in the infant from six months onwards. Out of a seething mass of feeling, a baby's mind evolves through a process of splitting between the good breast and the bad breast. If its desires are met, all is well with the universe and the baby relaxes in its omnipotent phantasy that it has created the object that meets its needs. If its desires are not met, the 'badness' is introjected into the emerging self of the baby – the baby experiences negative feelings and phantasies that come from the external object, the breast, and come to believe this about their self. A baby might think, on some unconscious level, 'I am hungry. I am not fed. The breast that feeds me is not enough. It is a bad breast. *I am bad*. The universe is an abyss'. As the baby tests its reality, there comes a point where it attains the depressive position and recognises the mother as a three-dimensional object or person who is neither all good nor all bad.

The importance of play

Klein saw these forces at work as she observed children at play. Play for a child is a very serious and savage business, and by it they offer a glimpse through the window of their mind. Our psychic life becomes a dynamic movement, backwards and forwards, between the paranoid-schizoid and the depressive positions played out from womb to tomb (Waddell 2002). Later writers have refined this by identifying other 'positions'. Ogden argues for an autistic contiguous position (1989) as a sensory baseline for all subsequent experiences. Other developments have included a transcendent position (Grotstein 2007) and a contemplative position (Black 2011). Klein invented the term 'projective identification' to explain how these early positions are recreated in the therapeutic space. Working with projective identification is an important skill to develop, one to which we shall return in Chapter 14.

Gavin's story

This is the story Gavin told me, sitting in my counselling room. Gavin kept getting into conflict with his Headteacher. Already head of an English department in a secondary school, Gavin found he despised the Head, and would make acid-laden comments in senior management meetings. The Head told him he had anger issues, which Gavin flatly denied.

I asked about his family of origin. An only child, Gavin grew up in an academic family where both parents were teachers (science and maths respectively). They drummed into him from day one that he needed to get to a prestigious university to secure his future career. As an adolescent, he spent all his time working, rarely mixed with friends, and was regarded as a loner. He gained extraordinarily high marks apart from his one hated subject, French, which drew his parents' ire. He felt 'Nothing was ever good enough for them' and, as an adolescent, was profoundly unhappy.

At the university he had always dreamed of going to, he found himself painfully alone. Everyone else seemed to make friends and be having a great time. Shy and socially awkward, he hid in his room, and he seemed to be doing the same in my consulting room, feeling much younger than his 35 years. As I sat with Gavin, I felt a profound sense of injustice, alongside a critical thought, 'Why did he allow himself to become so isolated?', mixed with feelings of anger about his passivity. One day, Anya, a girl on his corridor, knocked on his door and said, 'Gav, stop hiding and come for tea'. Gavin felt as if a bright light had been turned on in his dimly illuminated life. They started a relationship that lasted ten years, one that, as Gavin described it to me, seemed to be rich, fun, and fulfilling. Yet the cracks emerged and it finally broke down with Anya saying, 'You are always so angry with me'. Gav was perplexed as he said to me, 'I never get angry'.

Gavin reveals how we can use splitting and denial as a defence against the hate we feel for another in the paranoid-schizoid position. Unacceptable feelings get projected into others, which enable us to feel better. For Gavin, it is anger or rage that the therapist experiences as their own. Good supervision helps disentangle what feelings belong where and how these can be presented back to the client as their own. Klein's developmental schema focused exclusively on the inner world, while Anna Freud and Erik Erikson focused on balancing internal and external worlds.

Developmental lines and psycho-social stages

As a daughter, Anna Freud had the good fortune to have a loving, caring father (Freud and Freud 2014). He took her to Rome in 1923, despite his cancer diagnosis, because he so wanted her to experience this eternal city. He bought her a dog to keep her safe as she walked the streets in the evening. As an analyst wanting to discover her own mind, Anna had the misfortune to live in the shadow of her famous father. Yet, even within his looming shadow, she was able to grow and develop her own thinking. In parallel with Klein, Anna focused on child analysis. A qualified teacher, Anna established a school for the children of analysts in Vienna, then in 1941 the Hampstead War Nurseries for children, many made homeless by the bombing London endured during the War.

Taking psychodynamic therapy into the nursery pushes its practitioners to find new ways of researching and thinking about children and their families. In 1947, Anna Freud and Dorothy Burlingham started the Hampstead Child Therapy Course, followed by the Hampstead Clinic at Maresfield Gardens in 1951, becoming the Anna Freud Clinic after her death in 1982. Building on her experience as a child analyst, Anna believed there was one basic developmental line that served as a 'prototype' for all the others,

> which leads from the newborn's utter dependence on maternal care to the young adult's emotional and material self-reliance – a sequence for which the successive stages of libido development (oral, anal, phallic) merely form the inborn, maturational base.
>
> (Freud 1963: 254)

Anna adopted the metaphor of 'developmental lines' to show how the internal world and theory of mind created by her father needed, in practice, to take account of the external world in which the internal world grew, thus balancing object relations and ego psychology perspectives (Freud 1981; Edgcumbe 2000; Midgley 2013).

The idea of linking the internal and external world through a series of dialectical developmental stages in a psycho-social model was developed by one of Anna's analysands from Vienna, Erik Erikson (see Key Thinkers). Erikson's model was based on his analytic work and research including anthropological observation of native Sioux children in South Dakota. His subsequent books, *Childhood and Society* (1950) and *Identity and the Life Cycle* (1959), drew on this experience and outlined his thinking about a lifelong developmental process. Erikson outlined eight chronological stages of psycho-social development, each offering a challenge for our internal and external worlds (see Table 8.1).

Despite their linear chronology, in reality we move back and forth between stages, revisiting and repairing our psychological needs as required. Translating some of Erikson's stages, if all goes well our longing to be fully human encompasses: trust; a sense of self and autonomy; a desire to create; the experience of love and intimacy – physically and emotionally; and the ability to give and receive, with a sense of wholeness. Instead, we all too often encounter: broken trust; betrayal; shame; doubt that we are worth anything; guilt; inferiority; feeling trapped or isolated; stagnation; and despair. When things go wrong, each stage of our life reads like a disturbing Kafka novel, taking us into Kierkegaard's abyss and dread. Most of us live in-between, the place Erikson knew so well, in which, through an engagement with our inner and outer worlds, we find a balance.

Erikson's work enabled psychoanalytic ideas to be taken up in wider academic and therapeutic circles, holding together the inner and outer domains through the work of the

Table 8.1 Erikson's eight chronological stages of psycho-social development

Approximate age of development	Psycho-social challenges
Infant to 18 months	basic trust vs basic mistrust
18 months to 3 years	autonomy vs shame and doubt
3–5 years	initiative vs guilt
5–13 years	industry vs inferiority
13–21 years	identity vs role confusion
21–39 years	intimacy vs isolation
40–65 years	generativity vs stagnation
65+ years	ego integrity vs despair

ego. Erikson was influential in the newly emerging ego psychology and, in the words of one of his students, he 'made psychoanalysis come to life for the rest of the world' (Ross 1999: 648). Erikson's work enabled the real-world context to be taken into account in human development. For example, a refugee facing the loss of home, family, belongings, memories, and language, as well as the risk of exploitation and abuse, is left psychologically dislocated. They are at huge risk of declining mental health – new forms of psychopathology, self-harm, and depression. What has happened in the 'real' world changes what they can receive in their internal world (Volkan 2017) and what their children and future generations can receive in theirs (Alayarian 2016).

While developmental models have been superseded by more complex ideas tailored specifically to individual psychological, social, ethnic, and gendered contexts, Erikson made it possible to take ideas off the couch and out of the consulting room. Erikson's conception of the vital stage of 'basic trust' encapsulates many more complex psychoanalytic ideas, for example, and Donald Winnicott, to whom we shall turn next, continued Erikson's practice of moving beyond the clinical setting, advancing psychodynamic therapies into other health- and care-related disciplines (Kahr 2016).

Winnicott and Mahler – new developments

Donald Winnicott and Margaret Mahler took these complex psychoanalytic ideas forward. Winnicott did not offer a comprehensive developmental theory but his work, like Klein's, focused on pre-Oedipal developments in the internal object-relations world of the infant in connection to the mother (Winnicott 1960; Gomez 1996, 2017). Standing apart from Klein, Winnicott saw the vital importance of the internal world in connection to the external world, famously saying at a scientific meeting held by the British Psycho-Analytic Society in 1940 that there is no such thing as a baby. He later wrote that if you try to describe a baby, you always end up talking about a baby and another, such as a mother (Winnicott [1947] 1964). He evolved highly original concepts, such as 'true self' and 'false self', 'the holding environment', 'transitional space', 'potential space', the 'mother–infant matrix', the 'capacity to be alone', and the 'capacity for play' (Abram 2007). (The extent of Winnicott's work, the breadth and depth of his thinking, his innovation in clinical practice, and his ability to communicate is only now being fully realised with the publication of his twelve-volume *Collected Works* [2016].)

While Winnicott was informed by his experience as a paediatrician, he was still working with a paradigm that understood the infant through adult clinical data that was 'clinically reconstructed' (Stern 1985: ix). Mahler in the USA and Bowlby in the UK began to build bridges between psychodynamic thinking, infant observation, child psychiatry, and psychology. This is illustrated by the introduction to Mahler's best-known book:

> The biological birth of the human infant and the psychological birth of the individual are not coincident in time. The former is a dramatic, observable, and well-circumscribed event; the latter a slowly unfolding intrapsychic process.
>
> (Mahler et al. 1975: 3)

Separation and individuation are two distinct but overlapping developments. *Separation* is the infant's emergence from the necessary but symbiotic fusion with the mother. *Individuation* is the establishment of a distinct identity. Research supports the general validity of

Mahler's work but reveals the need to evolve this with newer findings from attachment theory (Lyons-Ruth 1991).

Summary

This chapter has barely scratched the surface of theories and research about how babies develop into adults. What it does reveal are the intricacies, richness, and diversity about how the psyche comes into being and how this shapes all human development. The more we can know, the better we are equipped to explore another's psyche, so all psychodynamic trainings build on these developmental understandings. My psychodynamic counselling incorporated a traditional Freudian Oedipal understanding; Kleinian good and bad breasts; Erikson's psycho-social stages (balancing the external and internal worlds); plus Winnicott's engaging and enigmatic ideas on a wide range of topics. (Many of these ideas were captured in Jacobs' influential book, *The Presenting Past* [1986, 2012].)

However, time marches on. As we become increasingly aware of the traditional Eurocentric approach of much therapy and are able to move beyond disputes about territory and institutional politics, we can challenge our comfortable and familiar narratives with newly emerging narratives.

Whereas here we have briefly looked at Klein, Anna Freud, Erikson, Winnicott, and Mahler, the next chapter engages with Bowlby, Stern, and a whole new generation of developmental theorists. Echoes of 'basic trust', the 'mother–infant matrix', and 'separation–individuation' resonate throughout attachment, as well as further advances in infant-observation research, which we will now examine.

Reflective questions

Thinking about your own psychological development, which theory do you most relate to?

Thinking about your clients or accounts of clients you have studied, which psychological theory are you most likely to use in practice?

Looking at research

Lyons-Ruth, K. (1991) Rapprochement or approchement: Mahler's theory reconsidered from the vantage point of recent research on early attachment relationships, *Psychoanalytic Psychology*, 8(1): 1–23.

Wang, Q. and Peterson, C. (2014) Your earliest memory may be earlier than you think: prospective studies of children's dating of earliest childhood memories, *Developmental Psychology*, 50: 1680–1686.

9

Learning from babies – attachment, the interpersonal self, and infant research

In this chapter, we shall examine further developmental theories that inform contemporary psychodynamic thinking and practice. These include Bowlby's work on attachment, Stern's multiple self-states, and findings from current research on how an infant grows and becomes a person.

My son was born on our double-bed at home at 6:00 am. This had not been planned. My wife experienced an unexpectedly rapid 45-minute labour, with the midwife arriving just five minutes before his entry into the world. As my wife was otherwise engaged, it became my responsibility to hold, bathe, and dress this small, quickening being, so alive and raw. I was deeply touched in ways I cannot put into words. I am in no doubt that babies enter into and have an impact on relationships from the very first moments of life. His eyes were fixed on me as I held him in one arm and gently bathed him with the other. All too soon, this idyllic scene was shattered. The discovery he had survived a short but brutal journey down a birth canal meant he was alive – and hungry. He released a piercing cry to let me know this, in case I was in any doubt. Immediately, he was a person with a self, a self that impinges on others physically, emotionally, cognitively, and relationally. This new person was attached to me immediately and remains so.

In the 30 years my son has been alive, the fields of infant development, developmental psychology, neurobiology, and neuroscience have revolutionised the way we think about how babies become people and learn how to relate. From their earliest moments, relationships matter. We know from our clients that they seek out psychodynamic (or integrative) therapy not because of problems they want to be solved, but to enter into a relationship where they are seen, can find a voice, and can discover meaning. The roots of our newer understanding of human personhood began with the empirical research of Bowlby.

Bowlby's attachment, separation, and loss – personal and professional

Bowlby studied psychology in his pre-clinical training at Cambridge, focusing on developmental psychology and evolutionary biology. Before resuming medical training, Bowlby worked in progressive schools and with maladjusted children where a colleague advised him to train as a child psychiatrist and psychoanalyst. His analysis was with Joan Riviere (also Winnicott's first analyst), a supporter of Klein who supervised Bowlby, but they fell out over how to work with children and he never completed his training as a child analyst. When he suggested new ideas on human development, he recalls becoming 'increasingly shocked by their intransigent attitudes' (quoted in Grosskurth 1986: 402).

Bowlby became convinced that babies were as much influenced by their external environment (and the quality of the relationships or attachments) as their internal world (where psychoanalysis often excluded the actual role of the mother). Working in a Child Guidance Clinic and later at the Tavistock, Bowlby's ideas developed, further shaped by the impact he saw on children of separation that took place because of the Second World War (separations that echoed his own in the First World War). Like Freud, Bowlby was passionate about psychoanalysis becoming a scientific discipline and made connections with ethology, systems theory, and cognitive psychology. Drawing on ethology (the science of animal behaviour), Bowlby found parallels in Harlow's experiments on rhesus monkeys, and his research on mothers and infants. Baby monkeys, like human babies, need not just nutrition to survive, but affectional bonds. Bowlby identified a baby's evolutionary capacity and biological necessity to engage with the mother, father, or the main adult caregiver as a form of attachment (Bowlby and Fry 1953). (This was later captured on film in Robertson's *A Two-Year-Old Goes to Hospital* [1951]. The film's emotive content, Bowlby's on-going work [1969, 1973, 1980], and further developments by Ainsworth [1969], greatly influenced childcare policies in the UK.)

Secure and insecure attachments

At its simplest, the nature of attachments could be secure or insecure. Insecure attachments can then be either avoidant, ambivalent, or anxious. (In 1986, Main and Solomon published research that added disorganised attachment as another category of insecure attachments.) Every person has a dominant early attachment pattern, which is a strong predictor of adult attachment patterns. Of great importance for psychodynamic work was the idea that an internal working model in the baby matched the form of attachment. To establish this, Ainsworth, Main, and colleagues developed the Strange Situation test and the Adult Attachment Interview (Kenny 2013). The test observes how one- and two-year-olds interact when different adults come and go, including the mother, father, and a stranger. The child's responses were identified as: proximity and contact seeking; contact maintaining; avoidance of proximity and contact; resistance to contact; and comforting. These indicated a form of attachment and a distinctive internal representation that Bowlby saw as an internal working model. These were mental representations, both of the other person and of the self, that shaped future relationships. It is these internal working models that dynamic therapy works with (Allen 2013).

Bowlby found an antagonist in Klein. Despite disagreeing with Anna Freud in some theoretical areas, Bowlby and Anna Freud maintained a cordial relationship (Freud 1960; Midgley 2013), yet he was dismayed by psychoanalytic politics. His work was dismissed because he did not offer a theory of mind, or deal with sexuality, Oedipal or otherwise. He withdrew from the psychoanalytic world.

Bowlby (1989) always believed he followed in Freud's scientific footsteps and that psychoanalysis would engage with research; however, his ideas were instead taken up by developmental psychology. While Holmes brought Bowlby to a wider therapeutic audience (2001, 2010, 2014), Fonagy and Target have taken attachment theory forward.

Fonagy has been the driving force, combining his work as a developmental psychologist, researcher, and psychoanalyst, as brought together in his seminal *Attachment Theory and Psychoanalysis* (2001). Fonagy and Target (2003, 2007) identify the psychoanalytic critiques of attachment but offer ways in which these can be re-framed and addressed, underpinned by empirical research (Daniel 2006). They demonstrate how understanding therapeutic interventions, client attachment styles, and therapist attachment styles can lead to better working alliances being formed and improved forms of attaching and relating for clients, although further research is required. Bowlby, building on Ainsworth's concept of the mother or caregiver offering a 'secure base' (1988), believes this can be replicated in therapy, or repaired if damaged (Heard et al. 2012). Fonagy and colleagues have also taken attachment theory forward through the development of mentalisation (Bateman and Fonagy 2004, 2016; Allen and Fonagy 2006) and its application to trauma (Allen 2013). Mentalisation is the capacity to understand the mental states of oneself, and the other. It is how we might imagine what the other person is thinking or feeling, along with what we might be thinking or feeling, as well as reflecting on the reciprocal relationship between the two. Fonagy argues it is the capacity to mentalise that is missing, lacking, or damaged in clients described with a borderline personality. It is an aspect of the self that normally emerges out of primary object relating and interpersonal experiences. Through a secure relationship with a responsive caregiver, the capacity to mentalise becomes possible. The infant uses the mother as a 'mirror' that first accepts their unprocessed feelings and then transforms them so they become reflected back as thoughts. This form of communication enables the infant to see, hear, and feel and, if necessary, to regulate their affective states as they become recognisable. They learn about shared thoughts and emotions and the impact on each party. If they do not learn, or do not have available someone who can show them this form of communication, things can easily go wrong, as the infant will find the understanding and communication of emotion like a foreign language. Attachment theory therefore offers a constructive approach, integrating the evolutionary and biological aspects of human nature with early interpersonal encounters, which helps establish internal representations and capacities, such as mentalisation, that are a vital foundation for healthy psychological development (Golding 2007).

In the UK, a parallel development that also drew on observing mothers with babies came from Esther Bick. Bick, whom Bowlby had asked to lead the child psychotherapy training at the Tavistock Clinic in 1948, pioneered infant observation. From her observations, and her unique concept of 'psychic skin' (1968), which we will explore further in Chapter 13, she found confirmation of a Kleinian view of development. Bick's ideas about how the skin acts as a container for the emerging psyche were further developed by Anzieu (1989) and Ulnick (2007) and applied to the contemporary desire for body modification (Lemma 2010). One Italian neurophysiologist and psychoanalyst, Mauro Mancia (2006), explored the idea that psychic development matches physiological development in utero. The mother–foetus relationship creates 'a container that might ensure the formation of an internal space in the foetus, adequate to the organizing of the Self' (Mancia 1981: 354). This self is present before birth and enables the baby to survive whatever traumas, both physical and psychological, the birth process brings. In the USA, developmental psychologists with analytic interest, such as Stern, Beebe, Emde, Lachmann, and Tronick whose work we now examine, have also taken up the important challenge of observing mothers and babies.

Stern's interpersonal self

Watching how babies interact with the world and those around them is fascinating. As their wide eyes gaze back at you, you wonder what is going on in their tiny minds. When they smile at you, their whole face is transformed, which triggers something deep within, possibly maternal/paternal feelings, or just a surge of warm emotion. In that moment, you are transformed from being an observer to a participant in their evolving world.

Daniel Stern was a developmental psychologist and analyst whose ideas grew out of observing infant–parent interactions (Emde 2013). Stern felt he inhabited two worlds – adult and child. He recalled understanding babies at the age of seven and being surprised that adults did not do so. He wondered if this bilingual capacity is something that gets lost in adulthood. In connecting this capacity to his own experience, Stern wrote,

> As an infant, I spent considerable time in the hospital, and in order to know what was going on, I became a watcher, a reader of the non-verbal. I never did grow out of it.
>
> (1985: ix)

Stern grew up into a skilled observer, commentator, and originator of the multiple selves found in the human psyche. The dilemma that Stern faced was making sense of people in the consulting room through psychoanalytic theories that did not fit their experience, where his formulations all began to sound the same. As he wrote,

> Yet the people were very different . . . The earliest months and years of a life held a firm and prominent place in the theories, but occupied a speculative and obscure role in dealing with a real person. This contradiction has continued to disturb and intrigue me.
>
> (1985: viii).

Stern's research drew on the same foundational idea advanced by Bowlby, that babies have an innate system motivated by survival that is relationship-seeking and is as powerful as any drive for sex or attachment. It is as if their brains are hard-wired and this is something they automatically do. This proposition had been advanced earlier by Fairbairn, a pioneering psychoanalyst, who highlighted the primacy of object-seeking (Fairbairn 1944; Sutherland 1989; Scharff and Scharff 2005). However, Stern offered empirical evidence to support Fairbairn's hypothesis, and further developed Fairbairn's concepts, putting forward his own idea of 'innate interpersonal relatedness' (1985: 128).

Stern's evidence-based practice was supported by videoing babies with their mothers from the ages of two, four, six, nine, 18, 24, and 36 months and analysing these videotapes, second by second, to trace the interactions between the mother and the baby as they developed into a child.

Continuous development and self-states

In contrast to Freud and Erikson, who thought about development in terms of stages, Stern saw development as *continuous*, with a person evolving different senses of the self. Stern's evolutions of the self unfold and overlap along with the normal physiological, cognitive, and emotional developments common to the first two years of life. Similar to Klein, Stern believed we move backwards and forwards in the development of multiple self-states.

While physiological and cognitive developments occur at key ages, which seem like stages, Stern wanted to avoid the rigidity of the forms of psychological development he saw in earlier phase or stage models. Stern's sense of the self consisted of the following domains of relatedness, acknowledging the importance of their context.

1. *Emergent self (birth to two months)*. Stern observed that before two months, babies can make direct eye contact, smile and make pleasurable noises, and take in the sights and sounds of their external environment. To do this, Stern argued there must be a rudimentary sense of self, contained in their mind.

2. *Core self: self with other, and self versus other (two to six months)*. The discovery of a further sense of self, a core self, enables the infant to interact with others. A baby can evoke powerful feelings in others attracting their gaze, smiles, and attempts at baby-language with a sense of excitement and enjoyment. This affirms a core self of relatedness, of being alive in the eyes of others, that through repetition they become familiar with. The baby and the mother's subjective worlds are joined in a mutual affirmation of both.

3. *Subjective self (7–15 months)*. The infant comes to understand they have a mind and other people have minds too. At a basic level, this can be shared and so begins emotional and subjective forms of communication, as well as the formation of intersubjective relatedness, which becomes the 'existential bedrock of interpersonal relations' (Stern 1985: 125). There now co-exists a core sense of self and a subjective sense of self, which interact together from the capacity for profound intimacy. If all goes well, a baby acquires the foundations it needs for all future relating. If all does not go well, these foundations can subside, unable to bear the weight of relating, and can be experienced as a form of abyss or psychic isolation, which Bion called 'nameless dread'.

4. *Verbal self (15 months onwards)*. The arrival of language gives the child a growing capacity to interact with others, for sharing their mind, feelings, and emotions and beginning to sense the thoughts and feelings of others, even if unable to understand. For the first time, they construct a narrative of their own life, expressed in the thought forms available to them at that age. Language offers scope for creativity and, in the developing mind, the capacity for symbolic thought.

5. *Narrative self (30 months onwards)*. In 1998, Stern made this addition. The capacity to tell others our narrative has huge significance for personal development, personal relating, and overcoming difficulties. It is a vital skill for the therapeutic arena. Therapists help their clients tell their narratives, discovering new untold stories as they are revealed. Psychodynamic therapists elicit the unconscious narrative in the client's story through transference in becoming seen 'as if' they are actors in the evolving drama taking place on the stage of the psyche.

Accompanying each new sense of self, Stern believed were 'representations of the interactions that have been generalised' (RIGS) (1985: 110). An infant or child builds up ideas and feelings about themselves through repetition. Children build an internal picture of the emotional world that acts as a template. Like Bowlby's internal working models, these become repeated in later interactions, in what Stern calls 'evoked companions'. Stern later refined his thinking to encompass what he called 'emergent moments', or 'moments of meeting', that exist within each stage of the self and contribute towards healthy interpersonal experiences (1995, 2004). Although Stern was criticised for rejecting Mahler's symbiotic phase, which we saw at the end of the previous chapter, she met with him regularly and was excited by these developments and the possibilities to stimulate and enrich psycho-dynamic thinking.

We have come a long way since Freud first proposed his psycho-biological model of development based on innate drives. Disruption or non-completion of psycho-sexual stages, or negotiating from one position to the next, leads to anxiety that emerges in the internal world of the psyche, but becomes expressed as symptoms in the adult experi-ence. A broader perspective now balances the internal world of the psyche with actual events in the clients's external world where reciprocal attachments and the formation of internal working models enhance our psychodynamic understanding of the formation of the self.

Important gains were achieved by moving beyond the consulting room – where early psychoanalysts did most of their observation and generated most of their insights –into the nursery or healthcare clinic. This inclusive step drew in a wide range of developmen-tal theorists and healthcare professionals. Given the evolution of the self as a category of meaning throughout the twentieth century, Stern's interpersonal approach, multiple self-states, and overlapping subjectivities revealed how we could grow into being a dis-tinctive person with a unique story. He offered a developmental map that fitted the contours of the late twentieth century and, more importantly, revealed a path for many others to follow.

Contemporary ideas from infant research and development

From 1995 onwards, a new generation of developmental researchers took up Stern's ideas. An important group, of which Stern was a member, emerged in Boston, which became known as the Boston Change Process Study Group (BCPSG) (Stern and the BCPSG 2006). Building on existing developmental models, they focused on how these influence the therapist–patient relational encounter (BCPSG 2010). Beatrice Beebe, one of Stern's research students, focused on minute mother–infant interactions (Beebe et al. 2016). She saw these as co-constructing our earliest relationships, including the development of a psy-chic structure in the baby (Beebe and Stern 1977; Beebe et al. 2005).

In Europe, Bråten researched pre-verbal communication with infants connecting to others and developed ideas with Trevarthen. Neither had links with psychoanalysis but they applied their findings to social and therapeutic contexts (Trevarthen 1974; Bråten 2007). Developmental researchers initiated new forms of understanding that enhance our understanding about the process of psychodynamic therapy.

New developmental research and contemporary psychodynamic therapy

What is distinctive about the 'new' research, represented by the developmental research of Beebe (and colleagues) including the BCPSG, is that they are not trying to evolve overarch-ing models. They apply their research findings to existing psychodynamic thinking and see what emerges in the creative outcome of such a dialogue. They recognise the significance of new ways of working and being with clients, based on the findings of infant development supported by neuroscience. These ideas are vital for developing specific skills in psychody-namic therapies, skills seen in the various vignettes up to now and in Chapters 13 and 14. The counselling room can become the nursery once more, with the opportunity to do something new but without encouraging regression or infantilising the client. The opportunity is to evoke, repair, or replace an earlier developmental life held in the unconscious, implicit memory, symbols, language, and embodiment of the client. These emerging ideas overlap and together form a creative synthesis. They represent the dancing landscape of contemporary developmental ideas offering the potential for further insights and discoveries. They enable the needs of the 'baby' still alive in the mind of the adult to be met. Any creative synthesis requires a unique combination of ideas and elements to form a connected, psychodynamic whole.

A creative synthesis – five key ideas

This creative synthesis of the psyche is built on five key ideas drawn from the newest research on infant development.

First, *babies are not passive bundles* to be passed round for admiring glances from family and friends. They actively interact from birth. Putting fantasy aside, babies interact and create experiences. They smile, sigh, gaze, relax, and evoke feelings in those observing or holding them. Many of these interactions are non-verbal, meaning pre-language – as a baby crying is pretty vocal and a powerful means of communication!

I was sitting in the café of an Italian delicatessen in Edinburgh one weekend. It was full of mothers, nannies, babies, and toddlers. A baby was crying, but not being heard. The carer was ignoring it. The baby cried even louder. I thought to myself, 'Will someone please pay attention to that baby', not because I wanted the peace and quiet, but because this baby was telling somebody something really important. As time went on, I found it almost unbearable. In part, this must reflect an early unconscious memory emerging into consciousness. You could say that in the timelessness of the unconscious, I was that baby. I had time to reflect and it made me wonder if there was something going on in my life that I was ignoring or not listening to. Beebe's work identified these early interactions. Close attention to mothers and babies shows miniscule changes in the face, body, and voice revealing fine graduations of meaning and mutual influence that normally go unnoticed by both mother and baby.

'Chase and dodge' were the terms given by Beebe and Stern (1977) to a specific pattern of mother–infant interaction described and illustrated through frame-by-frame photographs between a mother and her four-month-old baby (Beebe et al. 2016). What begins as a mutual gaze changes as the mother moves closer and the baby looks away or 'dodges' her gaze, thus avoiding the mother. The mother interacts to capture her baby's attention, or 'chases' them. Further avoidance can effect sadness in the mother. If this pattern continues, the mother shows her disappointment, looking away. If the baby copies this and also looks away from the mother, both become disappointed. The baby further withdraws by slumping into a collapsed posture, leaving the mother upset, possibly angry and the baby sensing a 'profound withdrawal' (Beebe et al. 2016: 130). All this has occurred in a two-minute interaction and is a predictor of an insecure–resistant attachment. This is just one form of interactive behaviour observed by Beebe and colleagues. There are many other behaviours that illustrate, to paraphrase Winnicott, there is no such thing as a baby, there is always a baby and an 'other'. Similarly, there is no such thing as an infant, there is always an infant and their interactions with an 'other'.

Second, research has demonstrated *the power of non-verbal communication as a key factor in interpersonal experiences and forms of attachments.* Trevarthen's idea of intersubjectivity is based on how powerfully infants relate to those around them, seeking out relationship, companionship, and initiating intersubjective existence (Trevarthen 1974; Bråten 2007). As Trevarthen explained,

> [In] conversations with a two-month-old [we encounter] the infant as a person seeking conversation, a person who is also interested in discovering experiences to explore and to 'talk about' with others.
>
> (1974: 25)

Trevarthen's 'primary intersubjectivity' is the capacity of the central nervous system, activated by the brain, to take in stimuli and transform these into actions such as eye contact, sound, movement, sucking, grasping, and holding, all activities that become a normal part of the life of a baby. These activities become a powerful means of interaction between infants and mothers/caregivers, hence the desire for 'conversation'. Trevarthen argued that babies are looking for forms of companionship and relationship that go beyond attachment and includes the desire to experience fun and play. The longed-for companions include mothers, fathers, grandparents, other adults, a twin, triplet, or siblings. Trevarthen therefore widened the scope of influence beyond the mother–baby dyad.

There is a strong correlation between these relationships and intersubjective experiences that lead to the later development of the person, for good or ill. Such developments can be re-experienced in psychodynamic therapies that focus on the intersubjective nature of experience and pay attention to key tasks, such as attunement, and the creation of an empathic bond. The failure of parental attunement and the presence of misattunement are key factors in later psychopathology, which Beebe (2000) links to Winnicott's idea of impingement. This arises through environmental failure and halts the development of the self and the continuity of being (Winnicott 1956), resulting in a false self and feelings of being 'unreal, futile (later bad)' (Winnicott 1955: 25). Guntrip (1969) developed his understanding of the schizoid experience as an early impingement that freezes the self, yet with a longing and waiting to be defrosted.

Third, *developmental research converges around relatedness and mental representations*. Drawing from Bowlby, Stern, Beebe, Lachmann, and Fonagy, the idea of some form of internal, mental representation explains the link between early attachments and later development.

> They have both predictive and interpretive functions – in both the emotional and cognitive domains – that direct processes of selective attention to (emotional) stimuli, perception of threat, defensive functions, and self-perception, among others . . . are capable of being brought into conscious awareness . . . in the course of psychotherapy through processes of self-reflection and mentalising.
>
> (Kenny 2013: 173)

These mental representations give a basis for intersubjectivity. By this, I mean the interaction between two people who possess different subjective senses of themselves, others, and the world in which they exist. When two people meet in therapy, the focus of their work is discovering the other, whilst avoiding recreating earlier impinged relationships, unhelpful attachments, and false-self experiences. So the person has a profound sense of 'I can be with an other because I have a sense of who I am. I am not merged with the other, nor am I totally independent and live in isolation from others'. Clients and therapists have their own mental representations, some that we are conscious of and some that are unconscious, or pre-conscious, waiting to be discovered, evoked through encounters in the therapeutic space. This forms the building blocks for intersubjectivity.

Fourth, *intersubjectivity offers the possibility of mutual dialogue and recognition* (Lyons-Ruth 1999) that prepares for a 'moment of meeting'. While traditionally psychodynamic thinking has been built around therapeutic encounters through transference, countertransference, projection, and projective identification, there are also 'now moments' and 'moments of meeting'. You get a sense of such a moment as a therapist when something intriguing happens with a client, or when they act in an unexpected way that is difficult to define. We either ignore this or respond differently and enter into an authentic moment of meeting and a new intersubjective connection is created establishing a co-created implicit relationship. One way of understanding this, advocated by Stern, is that moments of meeting form 'the nodal event in this process because it is the point at which the intersubjective context gets altered, thus changing the *implicit relational knowing* about the patient–therapist relationship' (Stern et al. 1998: 913).

Stern's understanding of moments of meeting offers a foundation for the intersubjective encounter in dynamic therapy, a theme we shall return to in Chapter 14. Moments of meeting have been further developed by the BCPSG based on new observation studies (2010). Bruschweiler-Stern adds a wider bodily dimension to moments of meeting, including the father, as part of this vital constellation in which an infant becomes a self, but cautions 'whether a meeting is achieved can be the beginning of the spiral – either positive or negative – that may become a characteristic pattern of relationship' (2009: 79).

Such moments of meeting also offer the opportunity for new implicit memories to be established, thus enabling the person to find new ways of relating, and in this regard therapy can have a vital part to play. This approach finds parallels between moments of meeting, coming as it does from a developmental observation context and Ehrenberg's (1974, 1992) concept of the 'intimate edge' found by reflective practice on the clinical encounter.

> By 'intimate edge' I mean that point of maximum and acknowledged contact at any given moment in a relationship without fusion, without violation of the separateness and integrity of each participant.
>
> (1974: 424f.)

Grounded in clinical practice, Ehrenberg provides an example of how allied concepts from infant observation and clinical reflection can be utilised effectively in day-to-day therapeutic practice.

Fifth, *implicit relational knowing is crucial for understanding how infants develop emotionally* (Lyons-Ruth 1998, 1999; BCPSG 2010). Observing the minute interactions of babies with those around them reveals that infants develop non-verbally and non-symbolically with some form of relational knowledge held in implicit memory (also known as non-declarative or procedural memory) that begins in utero. They bring this to interactions with those close to them, most often their mother or caregiver, becoming a dyadic form of consciousness and a pattern for all relationships (Tronick 1989). Implicit relational knowing, once established and supported by good attachments, is a predictor of positive mental health and interpersonal functioning. Conversely, implicit relational knowing and disorganised or ambivalent attachments predict difficulties in mental health and interpersonal relationships (Tronick and Beeghly 2011; Kenny 2013). It is a way of knowing something without knowing how or why you know it and is essential for all personal interactions. Therapists and clients bring into the room a vast repertoire of non-conscious experiences of so many others. These get expressed in their body, gaze, and tone of voice. These are intuitive moments of moving towards and backing away from. No words get spoken, and thoughts and emotions are forgotten in the profound meeting of the now that links with the unconscious but present internal patterns (Seligman and Harrison 2012).

The significance of these five key ideas taken from contemporary infant research and applied to dynamic therapies is that they inform us how mothers, fathers, and caregivers help babies develop a sense of self and form the basis for healthy psychological growth. If these development processes are missing, interrupted, or inconsistent, this potentially leads to psychological distress and dysfunction. Such distress can be experienced as a failure to develop an understanding of the self as likeable or loveable. An analogy taken from astrophysics is the term 'black hole' – where the laws of physics no longer fit and get distorted. In such a place, a person senses that in their psyche they are consumed by darkness (Ross and Loly 2013).

Integrating insights for effective practice

Ani's story

Ani (an Armenian girl's name meaning unique, beautiful, and exotic) felt anything but unique, beautiful, or exotic. Struggling with an eating disorder, Ani did not see herself in the mirror as others saw her in real life. She had striking eyes, held in an elegant oval-shaped face, with long lustrous black hair. Now in her early twenties, she had struggled with her weight for a decade. This had meant withdrawing from university much to her parents' disapproval. Both parents were busy academics. Pursuing their careers had meant frequent moves at considerable emotional cost to their only daughter, who was always given the best private schooling available. Ani recounted, 'We didn't do emotion in our house. You just put your head down and got on.' She recalled her father saying, 'Hard work never killed anyone'.

Her mother had what Ani now saw as undiagnosed depression, following her birth. It became clear that a failure in the early mother–baby interaction led to many later difficulties.

Ani's weight reached such a dangerous level there was a risk to her life, and she was admitted to a specialist in-patient unit. Within this service, a psychodynamic approach was used, and this enabled Ani to discover a sense of self, to put on weight, and to be safely discharged (Ross and Green 2011). The particular psychodynamic skill used was working with Ani's psychological defences against the unbearable pain of not being seen, or valued, somatised in her battle with her body. Containment through regular and consistent therapy enabled Ani to realise she did not have to control everything to feel safe.

Follow-up revealed she still struggles but is happier than before and has been able to return to university.

If Ani's case is viewed from the perspective of these key areas taken from contemporary infant research, the following story unfolds:

- First, depression and the 'dead eyes' of her mother, as Ani experienced it, left her feeling robbed of those minute interactions where the mother responds to the infant, rather than the infant meeting the needs of the mother.
- Second, Ani felt all conversations with her parents were transactional, not a form of communication through which they could form an empathic bond.
- Third, Ani's internal mental representation of herself was as barren and empty, and this was powerfully re-enacted through her relationship with food.
- Fourth, Ani experienced little mutual dialogue. She felt it was all one-way: 'I am seen if I am clever'; 'I am seen if I am hard-working'; and 'It is not acceptable to express emotions as these detract from the logic of rational thought'.
- Fifth, Ani wanted to be known but felt no sense of implicit relational knowing, only absence. Ani felt isolated and far from any intersubjective companionship. Her parents always felt remote and aloof. Ani had not learnt the social or emotional cues to be in relationship with others, hence school became problematic. Academically bright, Ani was adrift in a sea of adolescent currents, frightened by changes she was experiencing in her body. As the 'new girl', she found it difficult to fit in to existing groups. She learnt to be a social chameleon, blending in as a disguise, but with few real friends.

Therapists working with clients like Ani are able to draw on contemporary developments. But they can also benefit from parallel developments found in neuroscience, as we shall see in the next chapter. What psychodynamic thinking adds is what is going on in the inner and outer worlds. Early psychoanalysts and some traditional psychoanalysts today focus exclusively on the inner world of the psyche. What happens in a client's external world is only relevant in so far as it affects a world of internal objects symbolising early relationships, feelings, and events.

Relational psychoanalysis, psychodynamic therapy, and counselling (including those aspects included in integrative therapy) balance the inner and outer worlds of clients, finding correspondence between the two, through a process of intersubjectivity. In Ani's case, we can see the interweaving of the past and the present. The past reveals the mind and its representations of self, shaped by early parental (dis)engagement reflecting a bleak inner world. The present shows Ani's mind and body at war. Her mind is unable to accept she is worth taking care of while feeling out of control, the body becoming the battlefield for control that she must win in order to stop her sense of disintegration.

At first, Ani was unable to let good objects (people or food) nourish her. The containment of a therapeutic relationship and an in-patient context helped her re-establish boundaries. She slowly accepted that others wanted her to do more than survive, allowing her to become a self in a new way. Ani began to realise that she could absorb emotion and felt able to express that emotion to others instead of an angry and aggressive fight for control she turned in on herself.

Summary

Ani illustrates how many aspects of infant development research can be translated into therapeutic practice. As Green states,

Somewhere, equidistant between a transcendental optimism and nihilistic pessimism, there is the possibility that while damage from the past cannot be undone, new relationship experiences in the present, such as those afforded by a therapeutic relationship, can still effect changes.

(2003: 8)

This is the central hope of all of engaged in therapy. Yet what goes on in the therapeutic space also relies on what is going on in the brain. Matching the developments in infant observation and research, neuroscience has provided an illuminating range of findings that support these evolving ideas, as we shall explore in the next chapter.

Reflective questions

What does this new developmental research add to our therapeutic thinking and practice?

How would we know if such interactions were being repeated, or repaired, through our therapeutic engagement?

Looking at research

This chapter reveals the importance of research using infant observations of mother–baby interactions for psychodynamic practice. A demonstration of such work in action can be found in the DVD that accompanies the 2016 book *The Mother–Infant Interaction Picture Book* (Beebe, Cohen, and Lachmann).

10

Learning from our brains – infant development and neuroscience

This chapter identifies five discoveries from neuroscience that are of greatest relevance for contemporary psychodynamic therapy. We begin with the recognition of the different functions of the left and right brain and how these are influenced by therapy. We move to the nature of memory and how the brain structures memory differently, with consequences for how therapy works. We then examine how we learn through another person or persons, forming a dyad that enables self-regulation. We proceed to mirror neurons and the importance of developing empathic mentalisation. Finally, we investigative how the brain changes through relationships by incorporating the idea of plasticity.

The emergence of neuroscience and neuropsychoanalysis has huge implications for our understanding of unconscious processes (Solms and Turnball 2011; Solms and Leuzinger-Bohleber 2016). These advances Freud could only have dreamt of, yet not all psychoanalysts are enamoured with neuroscience (Pulver 2001; Blass and Carmelli 2007) and not all neuroscientists are enamoured with psychoanalysis (Ramus 2013). Neuroscience is a highly technical, complex, and conflicted discipline. For example, while some think that 'mirror neurons' offer definitive evidence that babies learn to experience and express emotion through relationships (Bråten 2007) and deficits in early parenting can be repaired through therapy (Gerhardt 2015), others are less convinced (Cook et al. 2014). Nevertheless, there is a growing consensus about the value of neuroscientific insights for dynamic therapies where the 'richness of the insights that have emerged from the work of Winnicott, Bowlby, Ainsworth and the attachment theorists integrates seamlessly with the work of Panksepp and Schore' (Wilkinson 2006: 4). From this immensely rich but diverse field, the five neurological developments we will explore emphasise the relational and intersubjective nature of the development of an individual as an evolving self.

The significance of neuroscience – the five key areas

Before we dive into the neural networks of the brain, which just like Alice in Wonderland's experience of going down a rabbit hole will be weird and wonderful, it is important to re-state why this is necessary. What happens in the room with a client draws on everything they and we have experienced, consciously and unconsciously. Each possess a brain that reacts, a body that remembers, a mind that recalls, and a self that requires connection. The nature of our ontological being and psychic reality stretches back to pre-birth when, from

28 weeks onwards, the earliest structures of the brain were established. From this point onwards, the brain becomes structured in a way that at some rudimentary level can process or record the experience of pain. Life begins and launches us on a journey of transformation or trauma – and invariably both, which therapy has the potential to repeat.

I first learnt therapy by growing up in a context where I now realise I was meeting the narcissistic needs of another person, at considerable cost to my own. This was not deliberate, just how it was, so in one sense I was 'born a therapist' involved in caring for others. Personal therapy helped me to meet my own needs, not vicariously live this through colleagues or clients. My initial experiential therapeutic training served me well enough, before embarking on formal training. What we know about who we are and what we bring into the room, including insights from infant development and neuroscience, becomes a vital resource in the therapeutic space.

So now let's go down the neural rabbit hole and, like Alice, see what amazing things we can discover. The brain is a mass of 100 billion interconnected nerve cells (neurons). Each neuron has two main branches: dendrites that receive incoming messages from other nerve cells; and axons that carry outgoing signals to other cells providing efficient, lightning-fast communication. Neurons communicate with other cells through electrical impulses. When a nerve cell is stimulated, an impulse moves to the axon and releases neurotransmitters. Neurotransmitters are chemicals that act as messengers, which pass through a synapse, the gap between two neurons, and attach to dendrites on the receiving cell. This process is repeated continually from neuron to neuron until the impulse reaches its destination. This is how the brain enables us to move, think, feel, and communicate.

Changes in any one of the myriad brain functions changes the way we experience our existence and how our clients encounter the world. For example, a sudden spike in our cortisol levels (a vital hormone produced by the adrenal gland) is usually caused by stress. Having increased levels of cortisol pumping around the body impacts on the metabolism and the immune system and increases blood pressure. Unbalanced cortisol levels are linked to how we regulate our thinking and feeling and are found in people suffering from depression, anxiety, anorexia, and various addictions (Gerhardt 2015).

Yet are we more than just the product of unregulated hormones? Can an addiction be just about what goes on in the brain? Answers to these questions can be found through examining the five key areas that link infant development, neuroscience, and psychodynamic understandings. These cover hemispheres of the brain, memory, self-regulation, empathic mentalisation, and brain plasticity.

The left and right hemispheres of the brain

The most accessible aspect of neuroscience for non-specialists to understand relates to the functioning of two hemispheres of the brain. Like all ideas that become popular, there are degrees of oversimplification, yet it works well as an explanatory metaphor that has a basis in what can be observed in behaviours and through the technology of neuroscience. We can better understand the complexity of communication and the development of intimacy in therapy by engaging with both hemispheres.

For the last forty years, Alan Schore (1994, 2001, 2003a, 2003b, 2011) has been integrating thinking from neuroscience, psychoanalysis, attachment theories, and many other disciplines. His thinking is wide-ranging, detailed, and complex, spanning four volumes as he delves into brain functioning and the influence this has on physical and emotional life. He influenced Gerhardt's *Why Love Matters* (2015), a helpful introduction to neuroscience and therapy. In the exploration of the self, which forms part of all good psychodynamic therapy, the right brain (and its connection with emotion) has a vital role to play in working with unconscious affect. We all fear disintegration, so when we see this emerging for our clients, they need us to enable them to go-on-being through our being with them. The implicit connection coming from our right brain, and theirs, offers a bond-of-being that is as powerful as what we say or do (Schore 2001).

This is of huge significance for the practice of therapy. Given the function of the left brain, short-term, goal-focused, cognitively based symptom-reduction forms of therapy have a vital place in the spectrums of therapies and many of these aspects are found in integrative forms of therapy. Yet given the function of the right brain, longer-term, dynamic therapies that encompass the experiencing body, address previous attachments, and are open to conscious and unconscious processes in a form of dyadic engagement, have a unique and vital place. McGilchrist captures this vividly:

> [The right hemisphere] yields a world of individual, changing, evolving, interconnected, implicit, incarnate, living beings within the context of the lived world, but in the nature of things never fully graspable, always implicitly known – and to this world it exists in a relationship of care.
>
> (2009: 174)

Contemporary psychodynamic counselling and psychotherapy offer that relationship of care. But we need both hemispheres. McGilchrist unconsciously parallels Winncott when he writes, 'there is no such thing as the brain, only the brain according to the right hemisphere and the brain according to the left hemisphere: the two hemispheres that bring everything into being also, inevitably, bring themselves' (2009: 175). He concludes his engaging work with the importance of the different hemisphere of the brain being able to offer different visions of who and what we are down through history including such dichotomies as the individual versus the whole, the transcendent versus the immanent, the general versus the particular, and estrangement versus belonging.

What we need is a good-enough understanding of both left and right brain for our work as therapists. For example, if a client has experienced an early trauma, the memory of this is stored in the right hemisphere of the brain at a feeling, affect-laden level. Talking and thinking, central to any 'talking cure', are the province of the left hemisphere. So a client, in telling you the story of a past event, in and of itself does not necessarily deal with any unspoken trauma if simply addressed cognitively or through a psychodynamic interpretation. The client needs to experience you, sensing your empathy, presence, and attentiveness in ways that trigger right hemisphere activity. Therapists who are unaware of this distinction could miss ways of unlocking the affect associated with such trauma.

The nature and form of memory

Our memories are vitally important to us. It is essential for therapists to understand this, especially as we are living in an ageing society with more and more people experiencing a loss of memory and identity triggered by dementia, which is estimated to affect 850,000 people in the UK today (Alzheimer's Research UK).

It has long been thought that our earliest memories date from the age of about three, though it is now thought to be earlier (Wang and Peterson 2014). Even so, such 'early' memory would not be from birth. Neuroscience has enabled us to see that there are different forms of memory and the processing of data (thoughts, feelings, symbols, words) that can be encoded and retrieved. The right and left hemispheres operate two different systems for recording and retrieving related to memory. The left 'brain' utilises explicit (or declarative) memory; the 'right' brain utilises implicit (non-declarative or procedural) memory, which is operative before birth but accelerates vastly after birth as its neural capacity grows.

> The earliest form of memory is unconscious, implicit, emotional, and inaccessible, arising out of the right hemisphere processing of early relational experience; it is online from birth . . . This memory system also stores emotional memory, which derives from emotional responses to stimuli . . . Negative or traumatic feeling responses are particularly associated with the amygdala. Appreciating the existence of implicit memory allows the concept of the unconscious to include anatomical structures where emotional, affective, sometimes traumatic, presymbolic preverbal experiences are stored . . . ready to be reassembled should they be required, but with the overlay of the most recent experience of remembering. Synaptic plasticity plays a significant part.
>
> (Wilkinson 2010: 29f.)

Such a memory system possesses 'plasticity', as do many other aspects of brain functioning, where the neuronal system can change as the result of new and different experiences. At one time, people thought babies were 'hard-wired' from birth, but such views have been superseded and research on the nature, storage, and recall of memory is in continual flux. While we need to be aware of new developments, it takes time to discover how such research applies to clinical practice.

Put in simple terms, the mind recalls everything, it is just that as we are not computers we do not have reliable data storage and retrieval programs. Yet it is still helpful to ask the question, 'What is your earliest memory?' Some clients cannot recall anything and what is repeated is commonly what they have been told or seen in a photograph or video. Others have very particular memories, often attached to a strong emotion experienced at the time. I have vivid memories of my third birthday on holiday in Millport, on the Isle of Cumrae in Scotland. I am standing on a beach ready to launch my new red toy boat. The sun burns down, the sky is blue, yet my wonder turns to despair when my little boat gets carried away by the waves. I start to cry, but thankfully some kind passer-by rescues the boat and me. However, I have no memory of being in hospital for a week due to an operation to remove my tonsils, aged five. Some people find that over time, 'flashes' of memory return. These again are often linked to powerful feelings, both positive and negative. This explains why we can see an image on a computer screen or in an art gallery that triggers a memory or a feeling, not always a conscious event, as well as an embodied sensation. As a teenager, I was visiting my grandparents in Glasgow and decided to go to the Kelvingrove Art Gallery and Museum on my own. Wandering around this place, which had positive childhood memories as a place of wonder, I encountered Salvador Dalí's painting Christ of Saint John of the Cross evoking my first mystical experience. I had a unique sense of time standing still, feeling the past, present, and future mingle together, swirling like a cloud revealing light and darkness, but a light and darkness that were within me. This was unusual and not a normal occurrence, then or now. Other people discover these connections in reading books. Words on a page do something to us. We can invest in the characters, plot, feelings or emotions, or thought processes, gaining new ideas, encountering different sensations as the mind spirals into other galaxies of thought, evoking a range of experiences all summed up by the phrases introduced in the first chapter – being alive and coming alive. The mind's capacity to think creatively by going beyond rationality, incorporating irrational and unconscious aspects of us, is a path to a transformed understanding. Through it we can glimpse something beyond, imagining freedom, wholeness, and connection.

Memory is a gateway to forms of imaginative transformation, part of all therapeutic work. In every session, there is the potential for the past to be present, if the therapist is attuned to affective states in their client, as well as able to interpret dreams, symbols, archetypes, and metaphors that come to life in a new way. (We shall return to the importance of memory and how it emerges in therapy especially when related to trauma in Chapter 12.) Given the importance of memory, psychodynamic therapists face a difficult challenge posed by clients with dementia. One of the 'sadnesses' of the ageing process is the onset of dementia characterised by memory loss.

Alf's story

Back in the 1980s, I visited patients on an acute dementia ward in a large Victorian psychiatric hospital. Such wards existed not just because of the decline of people's cognitive abilities, such as memory, but also because of the accompanying psychiatric disorders or dementia-related disturbances in behaviour. These included outbursts of rage and violence, profound depressions, paranoid delusions, and catatonic states. Locked into their own worlds, they fleetingly surfaced, and were gone again.

I recall visiting one patient, Alf, every week. We only ever talked about playing bowls (the hospital had its own bowling green). As I talked, Alf would interject the odd word, 'bowls', 'cigarette', and 'tired', and this seemed the extent of his spoken vocabulary.

Thinking of Alf helped me to reflect on what it means to be a person. Has their unique self become extinguished in their unquiet mind? The challenge is to find a connection, often in the distant past, that enables them to recover an experience of self as a person, while accepting the limitations of their current situation (see Phil's story later in this chapter).

'It takes two' – dyadic self-regulation and making meaning

Most people need another person to help them discover who they are. Winnicott's often repeated idea that there is no such thing as a baby, implying that there is always a baby and a mother, is true at the earliest stage of our development. We would not survive on our own.

I came home from my first day at school upset. When my mother asked me why, apparently I said, 'It's so sad. Nobody else has got a twin'. As I think about it now, I was externalising an internal feeling of my own sadness because Liz, my twin sister, and I had been put into separate classes. I recall looking out for her in the playground trying to find her, as a part of me. I didn't feel complete and it all felt surreal. This desire for the other, to connect, to be in relationship has its origins not only in the experiences observed by researchers in the first days, weeks, and months of life, but in the brain itself. Schore (2011) argues that a paradigm shift has taken place, which includes the neurobiology of unconscious emotion. The 'emotional revolution' of the last decade has overtaken the behavioural revolution of previous decades. There is a new emphasis on the development of the infant's neural networks and evolving orbitofrontal cortex. Mothers or caregivers act as external regulators of emotions and experiences in a way that has a profound lifelong neurobiological impact. If they do a good-enough job, the infant evolves a secure sense of self, expressed through healthful attachments, and has a mind that experiences being alive and able to make meaning.

How does this happen? Schore's four volumes cannot be compressed so readily but here is one indicative example taken from Gerhardt's reading of him.

> The orbitofrontal cortex does not just respond to other people and their emotional cues; it is involved with emotional behaviours. Connected to the amygdala, it quickly picks up on the emotion in facial expressions and tones of voice, but its role is more reflective: it considers what kind of response would be most appropriate and most likely to bring reward.
>
> (Gerhardt 2015: 54)

A baby seeks out others. It wants to be recognised, to be seen. The brain is active, intelligent, adaptive, and engages socially and emotionally though relationships. The gaze provides the greatest stimulus to the brain's growth and the baby's identity. When the baby sees a mother's dilated pupils, indicating their sympathetic nervous system is pleasurably aroused, the baby mirrors this response. Their heart rate goes up, and beta-endorphins and dopamine – which energises and stimulates and is linked to the anticipation of reward – are released in the orbitofrontal and prefrontal regions of the brain. So the gaze of a doting parent triggers brain activity and the production of hormones that enable the baby to feel connected and the social brain to come into being. Such developments enable empathy and a capacity to infer what others are feeling and builds foundations for all relationships.

We shall see later that therapy offers the opportunity for new insights into how we discover, feel, and control our emotions. When someone has been missing or is unable to provide external psycho-biological regulation, psychodynamic therapy offers the opportunity for a reparative dyadic encounter. We continue to learn to regulate what we think and feel through observing and taking in from others. How we experience, regulate, and express emotion is vital for healthy psychological development, and the absence of such internal regulatory mechanisms affect neural pathways. Some see in this the foundations of trauma-based injury, or the limited ability of the brain to adapt or be resilient when physical, sexual, emotional, or psychological injuries occur. This could include PTSD and borderline personality traits (Krause-Utz et al. 2014; Gerhardt 2015). In an intersubjective therapeutic encounter, the therapist relies on their client's and their own emotional dynamics and personality to guide the work. Schore adds another dimension by identifying a 'therapeutic affective encounter' (2001: 317f). This is where the therapist recognises their 'psychobiological state of mind and the counter-transference impressions made upon it by the patient's unconscious transference communications' (2001: 317f.). By paying close attention to points in the therapy where they sense increased affect, they can gain access to the client's internal working models and their most common transferential patterns, defences, and coping strategies for dealing with unwanted or uncomfortable emotions.

Schore (2011) goes on to argue that Freud's belief about the unconscious of one human being interacting with another's without engaging consciousness can be understood as a right-brain-to-right-brain communication through the relational unconscious of each other. Therapist and client influence each other, which is expressed through their behaviours and enactments. It is as if they get under each other's skin, right into the body, not just the mind and spirit. They think thoughts and feel emotions simultaneously or find themselves resisting this depth of engagement. Tronick (2007) developed a dyadic state of consciousness model that includes the conscious and the unconscious, arguing that when a dyad is formed, something greater comes about. Through dyadic encounter, there is a shared learning and something is created in the minds of the persons that together are experienced as being valued, discovering meaning and sensing an increased self-worth. In the intersubjective encounter, there is a continual flow of dyadic rupture and repair, each meeting re-enacting the childhood of the client, of which they are currently unconscious despite it being stored within a procedural memory system in the brain. From this, something qualitatively new emerges and one mechanism for achieving this is found in the activity of mirror neurons, empathic mentalisation, and brain plasticity.

Mirror neurons and empathic mentalisation

The discovery of mirror neurons has been hailed as offering empirical and scientific support for psychodynamic ideas. Mirror neurons were discovered through research on the neural representation of motor movements in macaque monkeys (Rizzolatti and Craighero 2004). It was observed that when a researcher picked up some food to hand it to a monkey, this fired motor neurons in the frontal and premotor cortex, the same neurons that would fire when the monkey grasped the food. So there was a form of neural anticipation through observation, matched by a form of neural reception that connected the researcher and the monkey. This result was replicated in monkey-to-monkey interactions and the first research on human mirror neurons in 1995. From this research, indicating a rudimentary capacity for empathy, therapists have made important links to the roles of attunement, emotional and relational communication, the place of empathy and how this shapes a person's psyche, and the development of the mind (Gallese 2003; Gallese et al. 2007). Although some argue there is not yet sufficient evidence for the existence of mirror neurons in humans, it is clear that this is a promising area of research (Ferrari and Rizzolatti 2014). From a psychodynamic perspective, mirror neurons enable implicit and explicit communication for mentalisation, attachment, and the development of empathy (Hooker et al. 2008). The BCPSG argue that mirror neurons, and other associated mechanisms, provide a neurobiological basis for the development of not just empathy but *intersubjectivity*. We can 'feel' what it is like to be the other person, imagining their pleasure, sadness, pleasure, or pain. We can respond to them in a way that affirms their feelings and allows them a sense that they are not going mad (always a deep-seated fear) and affirming their humanity. It can also form a building block for attachment patterns that develop between a baby and a parent or carer.

When an infant experiences distress, the caring, containing, holding presence of another person – be they a parent, carer, or other – validates the infant's experience of pain and prepares for the soothing encounter that ensues. All these helping people are using their system of mirror neurons to help them respond. The absence of such encounters leaves a baby distressed and ambivalently attached, which often prefigures greater relational difficulties in later life. Yet even worse may happen. If mirror neurons operate as part of an intersubjective system, there is the potential that the infant takes into itself the negative, damaged, depressed, anxious, or traumatised self-states they encounter in the caregiver. This could be one mechanism underpinning the inter-generational transmission of trauma and damaging self-narratives (Ginot 2015). The task of dynamic and integrative therapists is to work with the dynamic brain and dynamic unconscious of the person sitting in front of them in such a way as to facilitate a relational and intersubjective encounter. Bion (see Key Thinkers) captures this task in practice through his ideas of containment (Levine and Brown 2013). Unprocessed fragments of experience that are contained in the psyche are taken in by the therapist, as if in a mirror neuron activity of the psyche, processed, detoxified, and given back to the client. This has the potential to change the person for the better, as well as make up deficits or repair damage from the past.

Synaptic plasticity and the changing brain

Brain functions can change and are not hard-wired, as once thought. The term 'hard-wired', originally from computing, related to permanently connected circuits devised to perform a particular fixed function. It is commonly used to describe some aspects of brain function such as babies being 'hard-wired' to learn language – it is something they do without having to think about it. Most brain functions happen through unconscious processing and develop neural pathways or patterns and synaptic connections that influence actions, emotions, and behaviours. Neuroscientists discovered that these patterns or connections, rather than being hard-wired, could be re-routed or changed, hence the idea of plasticity or neuroplasticity. If neural pathways are blocked or not used for any reason, the brain is able to utilise new neurons and form new pathways, thus allowing new learning and remembering, intellectually and emotionally (Doidge 2008).

Our understanding of plasticity offers a key to unlock and understand the possibility of how minds change through the process of dynamic therapy. It is this idea that also underpins the contemporary focus on mindfulness (Williams and Penman 2011), which uses meditation as a way of influencing existing neural connections or potentially developing new pathways or connections. Williams and his research team (2014) have shown how mindfulness-based cognitive therapy can lead to a significant reduction in levels of depression, and is more effective than drug-based treatments for chronic long-term depression. Tang et al. (2015) correlate mindfulness and its beneficial physical and emotional effects with changes in brain states, whilst recognising more detailed research needs to be done to identify the neural mechanisms that bring this about. These are key examples of non-traditional psychodynamic skills in practice, bringing about key therapeutic outcomes.

A reminder of the importance of plasticity is that we know at the other end of the spectrum the consequence of neuro-rigidity. This is where neural pathways degenerate due to damage or the ageing process, resulting in Alzheimer's disease or forms of dementia.

Phil's story

Phil (in his sixties) was referred by a colleague. He was shy, nervous, and lacking confidence, almost apologising for seeing me. His story was that he had been looking forward to the freedom of retirement but, shortly after retiring, had the first of a series of minor strokes. He realised he was losing memory, and found himself angry, often feeling out of control. Emotionally, it was as if the filters he normally used had been switched off and he would say and do things he was later shocked about.

Working with Phil was going to be challenging but we arranged to meet weekly for ten sessions. On coming back each week, Phil had 'forgotten' much of the previous week's session. This made me realise how much we rely on building a relationship week by week while, on an unconscious level, me just being there every week did something for Phil.

When given permission to 'forget' and realising it did not lead to being judged, Phil found he could work with what he could recall and progress. Therapy in this context could never result in delaying what had been diagnosed as a degenerative process. It could, however, help Phil overcome the sadness he felt that his later years were not going to be what he had hoped for. Phil showed immense courage in facing this. In the process, we found ways of connecting with material from his past through symbolism and metaphor that sank deep into him in a way he was able to retain. The brain can change and the nature of the change is influenced by relationships.

Phil had been brought up to go to Church and, as a child, had listened to many Bible stories, including Jonah and The Whale and Daniel in the Lions' Den. When I used parts of these Bible stories as metaphors of his experience, he was able to grasp their message and remember them. Sometimes he would refer back to the previous week saying, 'Remember when I was in the lions' den?' This was a reminder of how important relationships are, not just as a baby when forming a sense of themselves through relational engagement, but in forging a changing identity in the face of dementia. It is also a reminder that our clients bring with them the tools to unlock their situation if we are able to work with them. A deep listening to Phil allowed me the opportunity to align my therapeutic tools with his. Phil presented the tool of stories from the Bible learnt as a child. In revealing this aspect of his past, I was able to bring the past into the present – a key psychodynamic idea – allowing the client's unconscious associations to emerge in new ways.

Summary

This chapter adopts an interdisciplinary approach that finds great value in recent developments in infant research and neuroscience. This has been applied to psychodynamic thinking and clinical practice, though this is only the start of an on-going process as we learn more. Psychodynamic and integrative therapists are united by a desire to bring, at the very least, *help* and, at the very best, *healing* to those in need who long for a way out of the abyss of their unconscious and conscious trauma-driven worlds. Incorporating these new understandings of the brain enhances this task.

The next chapter deals with who we are as sexual and gendered persons, which profoundly shapes our experience of life.

Reflective questions

To which aspect of these new developments in neuroscience can you most relate in your work as a therapist or in your planned approach?

How do you envisage putting these ideas in practice?

Looking at research

Solms (1997, 2013) has pioneered this area, especially as applied to psychoanalysis. Working alongside colleagues such as Kaplan-Solms, Turnball, Panksepp, and Leuzinger-Bohleber, he has revised Freud's understanding of the unconscious in the light of empirical research.

Solms has widely publicised his ideas through on-line presentations, TED Talks, and YouTube lectures (accessed 28 October 2018). Other neuroscientific researchers who have attempted to popularise the subject in order to make it accessible to wider audiences include Schore (1994, 2003a, 2003b, 2011), Damasio (2012), and Siegel (1999, 2012).

11

Learning about sexuality, gender, and identity

The most powerful way our identity is shaped relates to our sexuality and gender. In this chapter, we begin with the importance of difference and diversity, which forms a vital part of contemporary psychodynamic therapy. We move on to Freud's understanding of Oedipus but go beyond this to discuss new developments showing how Freud was both a revolutionary thinker and a traditional patriarch, drawing on psychoanalytic feminist critiques of Freud that have shaped new understandings that best fit our experience today. Benjamin (1988, 1995, 1998) offers a radically new interpretation of the dynamics traditionally expressed through the Oedipus complex, but re-works these in a way that helps us in our work as therapists. We conclude with a brief examination of sex in the consulting room – although don't take this literally.

Difference and diversity

One way in which contemporary psychodynamic therapy justifies the name 'contemporary' is through a commitment to addressing issues of diversity and difference in the individuals we meet and the society in which we live (Wheeler 2006; Muran 2007). Therapy is set within a wider social context of static, binary, oppositional, and fixed understandings of gender and sexuality, and a move towards more fluid expressions of gender and sexuality (Lemma and Lynch 2015). Although writing about gender, Reisner sets the scene well by illustrating the complexity of the debate:

> Gender is a psychic conglomerate assembled from components that are conscious, unconscious, biologically determined, symbolically constructed, culturally normed; that drive, too, is a psychic construct, induced, relational, and conflictual; that the combination of and conflict among such sexual, generative, acculturative, destructive processes results in a limitless variation of gender identities, object relations, motivations, and practices. Psychoanalysis at its best is a process of discovery and recovery, rather than a prescription for normalcy.
>
> (1999: 1057)

These comments equally apply to sexuality. For therapy to be part of our future, rather than an expression of the present or a representation of the past, there is a fundamental social and political dimension it needs to regain. Only then can it escape out of the consulting room and onto the streets (virtual or otherwise).

Why is this necessary? Our clients, like ourselves, are deeply rooted in the contemporary world, a world that looks very different depending on where we locate ourselves. Invariably, we are shaped like wet clay thrown on a potter's wheel, by age, class, wealth, gender, sexuality, race, religion, ability or disability, and in many other ways. Yet different forms of clay also have an inherent plasticity in how they can be worked with. Our plasticity (in a non-neurological sense) is how we have taken the opportunities that have arisen in our life, overcoming defences and resistance to change, allowing risk to be familiar, entering into 'aliveness', and avoiding psychic forms of sleepwalking to conformity or oblivion. Often, however, clients come to therapy with many regrets regarding these opportunities.

Niall's story

Niall left Northern Ireland because of the 'Troubles'. He did not feel safe either as a Roman Catholic or as a homosexual man.

He came to therapy not to address a homosexual identity, which was healthy and secure, or because of any lingering religious guilt. As I listened, he communicated an existential form of depression that lurked just below the surface. I did not realise this immediately as Niall was lively, telling engaging and colourful stories of his past. Yet after each session, I felt drained and, as I explored these feelings in clinical supervision, my supervisor enabled me to identify the dynamic process of projective identification. This is where a client locates their split-off feelings in the therapist to the extent the therapist feels the unacceptable feelings the client cannot own. Bion saw this as a primitive form of communication that, once identified and worked with, can help emotional health and psychological growth.

We discovered Niall's depression was related to the early loss of his mother and being left living with a depressed alcoholic father. His loss was around who he was as a child, with no fixed pointers or people to guide him other than his one sibling, a much older brother. His brother also left to escape some unknown miasma that drained his soul but left Niall bereft and alone. He had no guides to help him understand his maleness, powerlessness, struggles with sexuality, alongside his numbing losses.

Niall's story illustrates the pervasive experience of loss, as well as the challenge to understand issues of gender and sexuality, individually and societally. Like Niall and his brother, we too have grown up in, and through, the soil of a society that has unique complexities and contradictions. At best, a country can unite around a cause, an event, and a vision for justice, equality, and inclusion, where people can fulfil their potential. At worst, it can divide and fracture, exposing deep prejudices and fears, often focused on someone who is different from me, the 'other', the scapegoat. They then become subject to derision, or as we have seen so tragically in the twentieth century, extermination (Friedländer 2007; Rees 2017).

Like identical twins, it is always difficult to separate gender from sexuality. Gender identity is a concept formed from two aspects of the self. Our core gender identity is based on our physical, embodied self-image, typically but not exclusively male or female. Along-side this is our gender *role* identity, which is how we see ourselves as masculine or feminine, in accordance with or in opposition to family, social, or cultural understandings. This links to our sexual identity, which is formed from four aspects of the self: our biological sex; our gender understanding (as discussed); our sexual behaviours (in fantasy or actuality); and potential for reproduction (in fantasy or actuality). In most cases, a settled sexual identity is established during and following puberty, although this can change, and is expressed though fantasy and the desire for or avoidance of physical sexuality. Clearly, there is a healthy overlap as both are central to our identity, which we can now explore in the fol-lowing sections. We begin with Oedipus, before turning to gender, then sexuality.

Focusing on Oedipus

In Freud's study, on a wall behind his desk, hung a black and white engraving of Oedipus and the Sphinx. In it a relaxed, muscled, naked Oedipus engages with the Sphinx, a fantastic creature composed of the head and rounded breasts of a woman, the body of a lion, and the wings of a bird. Little did Oedipus realise the traumas he was about to endure. Freud's collection of antiquities located throughout his study also contained several sculptures of the Sphinx laden with symbolic meaning about power and sexuality expressed within the female form. This classical portrait taken from Greek mythology represents Freud's titanic idea of the Oedipus complex as the shaping event that structures our experience of sexu-ality and gender.

How does it do this? While we examined this in Chapter 8, it is important to capture what Freud was doing with his concept before we further explore gender and sexuality. He took seriously the confusions, curiosities, pleasures, and fantasies of a child experiencing themselves in and through their bodies, and their feelings about parents or other parental figures. They are searching to find where they belong, and where they fit with a father and a mother (as Freud expressed it) in a tripartite structure (see Figure 11.1).

This experience included sexual rivalry with the same-sex parent, and sexual longing for the opposite-sex parent. Allied to a fear of castration, a metaphor for who holds power, the negotiation of this Oedipal complex between the ages of four to six leads to an under-standing of the prohibition on incest, awareness of familial and generational boundaries, and the formation of the super-ego. As we saw in Chapter 8, the Oedipus complex and its resolution orientate our experience of gender and sexuality in a binary fashion where gender is unquestioned and our sexual identity and aims are fixed. Males copy males, father and son, and no longer compete for a mother's love and attention, focusing their emergent

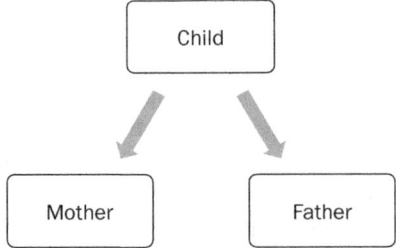

Figure 11.1 Freud's tripartite familial structure

sexual feelings, to become latent until adolescence, on a female of their choosing. Girls experience a similar pattern. All this makes sense in a heterosexual and patriarchal world – a view of the world that no longer fits with the clinical realities we meet every day. For example, therapists in university counselling services are reporting many more students working out where they belong and identifying as transgender. The Oedipus complex still engages us today because it speaks of something very powerful we have all experienced, even if the terminology has changed.

An often-overlooked aspect of the Oedipus story is his passionate desire for truth. It was this same passionate desire for truth (and justice) that led feminist and psychoanalytic thinkers, Mitchell (1974) and Chodorow (1989), as well as Lacan (Jones 1999), Deleuze and Guattari (1972), and Weatherill (2017), to challenge 'conventional' understandings of who and what we are as gendered, sexual beings understood from an Oedipal perspective. Psychodynamic therapies have been slow to think about, and respond to, the complex issues of gender and sexuality, although this is changing.

Focusing mainly on gender

Reisner emphasised how complex gender is, not least because it forms a vital part of our identity. Gender is not something we can be neutral about, evoking very powerful feelings, often unspoken. Tensions exist because some view gender as hard-wired (despite the advances in our thinking about plasticity), whereas others view it as socially constructed. This is one reason why trans-issues have triggered so much impassioned, if not inflexible, debate. We cannot deny the experience of on-going gender inequality, the persistence of patriarchal attitudes, commonplace discrimination, the limitations of binary thinking, and the invidious presence of sexual exploitation. Given there are no easy solutions, an important place to begin is how we come to understand whom and what we are as gendered, sexual beings.

If we turn to Freud for help, we hit a big problem that needs explanation. While the Oedipus story encapsulated Freud's thinking, it also severely limited it. At its most basic level, Freud's account of human nature is a story about how people go from being polymorphously perverse (pleasure-seeking from any source, as we see later in this chapter) to having a settled heterosexual identity – and the idea that if something prevents this from happening, it also prevents the development of psychic structures essential for healthy mental functioning. Put starkly, you could not be healthy or mature as a person if you were not heterosexual. While this sounds extreme to our ears, it was only in the late 1980s (and even later in some cases) that you would be accepted for psychoanalytic training if you identified as homosexual. This was because it was assumed you had not sufficiently resolved your Oedipal dynamics.

So Freud, as a male patriarchal figure of his time, took gender for granted rather than exploring it in any detail in his thinking. This chapter examines how a psychodynamic understanding of gender has changed since Freud's day.

Living in the shadows

Despite psychodynamic therapy's many strengths, the shadow side of an analytic heritage has been the sacrificing of people's experience as feminist, male, trans, gay, lesbian, and queer therapists before the altar of an Oedipal tradition and a theoretical orthodoxy. The dominance of a fixed landscape model of psychoanalysis has left gender and sexuality in the shade, hidden in the shadows for fear of rejection. The irony is that Freud's original and radical vision of sexuality that ushered in the twentieth century has evolved into civil wars in the profession about orthodox theories and practices. Fights over who is in control are of little interest outside analytic circles.

How has this come about? Historically, a person's stance on the Oedipus complex was a definitive mark of inclusion, or in Jung's case, *exclusion*. Why? Take one example. Traditionally understood, the Oedipal complex leads to the formation of the super-ego, a central component in Freud's understanding of the mind involving conscious and unconscious processes. To deny this is to challenge the entire edifice of Freudian ideas. Although Klein changed the Oedipal time-line with the super-ego present from the start of life outside the womb, she still adhered to the power of Oedipal dynamics that influence our basic conflicts about sex, gender, love, aggression, jealousy, rivalry, competition, narcissism, and reparation. Failure to negotiate the Oedipal complex processes therefore becomes a source of psychical malfunction that can be seen in various forms of adult psychopathology associated with these basic conflicts. Yet the traditional Oedipal focus on: the penis as the source of power; the lack of a penis for a girl; the fear of castration or abandonment; the assumption that that there is a gendered split between desire and identification; and the norm that healthful same-sex identification leads an opposite-sex love object – has rightfully been challenged by Barden (2006, 2015) and Gilmore (2012).

> For the girl, the effect reverberates throughout her personality, creating feelings of inferiority and deficiency and affecting superego formation . . . Modern psychoanalytic theory has radically revised these ideas, which seem deeply influenced by the zeitgeist of the time . . . the impact of feminism . . . has led to radical revision of much of psychoanalytic theory regarding female psychology with a recognition that the girl struggles with anxieties specific to her own body, her feminine identifications, and the variations of her superego injunctions in both universal and idiosyncratic ways . . . all of these conflicts leave their imprint on adult personality.
>
> (Gilmore 2012: 124)

Jessica Benjamin, a contemporary relational psychoanalyst, feminist, and social theorist, has offered a more nuanced way of understanding male and female identity that also adopts an inclusive approach to sexuality. Benjamin moves from Freud's static binary Oedipal stance to a dynamic process working with Hegel's ideas of the master–slave dialectic. This dialectic is elaborated in a story Hegel wrote about a master and a slave. The identity and function of the master depends on the existence and recognition of a slave who, in order to function as a slave, needs to supress their own identity and desires. The slave, by negating aspects of the self, can come to educate and transform that self and so be freed from slavery. Benjamin observes this dialectic is seen in all issues of gender, sexuality, and power. She argues there needs to be a move away from static power-based relationships to a fluidity and multiplicity of gender and sexual identifications enabling psychic enrichment throughout life. In one of Benjamin's key texts on gender and sexuality, *The Bonds of Love* (1988), she begins by identifying an impasse found in Freud's *Civilization and Its Discontents* (1930) where he locates psychoanalysis within a wider social context. She critiques Freud's vision of the tensions between instinct and civilisation, believing this created an impasse and obscured the crucial question of domination.

Freud has thus given us a basis to seeing domination as a problem not so much of human nature as of human relationships – the interaction between the psyche and social life. It is a problem that must be defined not simply in terms of aggression and civilized constraints, but as an extension of the bonds of love.

(Benjamin 1988: 4f.)

Benjamin focuses on the interplay between love and domination as a two-way process seeking 'to understand how domination is anchored in the hearts of the dominated' (1988: 5). For Benjamin, the mother–child dyad is as important in psychic development as any later Oedipal development – a fact supported by the extensive developments in infant research we examined in Chapter 9. This marks a shift from the Oedipal to pre-Oedipal and places the mother, rather than the father, at the centre of psychic development. It recognises a shift from drives and defences to egos and objects, seeing the emergence of the self vitally connected to the relationship with the other. So when a birth or adoptive mother holds a baby,

the mother who feels recognized by her baby is not simply projecting her own feelings into her child . . . She is also linking the newborn's past, inside her, with his future, out-side of her, as a separate person . . . she is certain and he or she is already someone, a unique person with his or her own destiny.

(Benjamin 1988: 13)

Yet this baby is still unknown to the mother, even if she has had children before, as each baby is unique and responds differently. A baby is a paradox, like and unlike any before or after, linked in a bonded sense of intimacy but always with a sense of otherness. Benjamin builds on the object-seeking dimension of each person that seeks out relationships, first and foremost with the mother (or caregiver). The mother offers a bond of love that remains within the psyche and is available to access when engaging with others. Fathers are also present and offer a different model of strength, a strength that is idealised but one that comes with the threat of dominance. A child longs to be loved with bonds of love and bonds of strength, where dominance is identified and avoided, and power and powerlessness are held in balance. This forms the foundations for later gender and sexual identity based not in any binary drive system but on a relational fluidity within a masculine–feminine continuum. Thinking more creatively about trans, we move beyond linear continuums with male–female polarities and trans as somewhere in the middle, neither one thing nor another. More creatively, we can think about strands of gender that intertwine and become woven together.

Benjamin's intersubjective approach argues that intrapsychic development requires the recognition of, and engagement with, our gendered and sexual self-representation. Benjamin balances mutual recognition with being uniquely one and alone, the two held in tension:

. . . when the conflict between dependence and independence becomes too intense, the psyche gives up the paradox in favour of an opposition. Polarity, the conflict of opposites, replaces the balance within the self . . . It also sets the stage for domination. Opposites can no longer be integrated; one side is devalued, the other idealized (splitting).

(1988: 50)

It is this domination, seen in the development of the baby and in adult erotic life, that gets played out in the spheres of gender and sexuality. Our paradoxical dependence on others for our own sense of self is the core of the problem: if we destroy the other, there's no one left to recognise us but there's no way of avoiding the danger that the other can destroy us. This is Hegel's master–slave dialectic at work, where our identity depends on the recognition of the other, which forms a central theme in psychotherapy. People come to therapy to discover who they are (although they would never have thought of themselves as master or slave) so they can more fully engage with others in a new way that does not subjugate but recognise who they are.

For Benjamin, the solution for the paradox of recognition is for it to continue as a constant tension we work and re-work throughout life. Radical equality comes about through a mutual recognition of the other as male, female, mother, father, attracted to and identified with the same and the opposite sex. Although Benjamin does not discuss this, it is important to add that siblings and twins also play a vital part in coming to understand how we are part of and separate from others in the evolution of our gender and sexuality (Mitchell 2003).

Bonds of love

People come to therapy looking for recognition and for help in overcoming 'bonds of love' that have been skewed in some way.

Karen's story

Karen cried about her father, a remote man she loved with a passion but who gave her so little. She was always unfavourably compared with her brother. Karen recalled getting her exam results and proudly showing him her 9 'A' grades and one 'C' grade, longing for some word of approval. He said, 'Shame about the "C" grade, you'll need to work harder'. That was it. No recognition of her as a loved, bright, intelligent girl. No bonds of love, as Benjamin sees it.

When Karen said those words, as a man I felt ashamed wondering how the father could so miss this opportunity to show his daughter love and approval. I felt tearful, sensing her abject shame, yet I also felt trapped in the power dynamics that so many men, women, and trans persons get locked into. At times like this, it is vital that one's gender as a therapist is part of a clinical supervision process so that we can avoid collusion, idealisation, splitting, transferential processes, or acting out unconscious dynamics. I, working in a contemporary psychodynamic context, needed to practise the skill of being aware of my gender role identity just as much as that of my client.

Contemporary psychodynamic therapy attempts to deal with some aspects of the ever-present tensions around gender and sexual identity (Lemma and Lynch 2015). It offers a way of moving towards mutual recognition, whilst working with sameness and difference, individuality and complementarity, power and powerlessness, alongside freedom and domination. These psychodynamic processes underpin all aspects of human relating. When we cannot bear the tension inherent in these dichotomies, we resort to the certainty of a fixed position that ultimately diminishes us and others – we become blind to the complexity of our contemporary social context and to the complexity of our and our clients' unconscious. It was for this reason Benjamin moved beyond an Oedipal understanding, arguing that the focus on the 'self' in contemporary culture has superseded Oedipus with Narcissus as the myth of our time. Nowadays, therapists frequently work with narcissistic disorders or pathologies of the self.

> [What is required is a] new Oedipus, the rereading of the story as a confrontation with knowledge of self and other, [which] holds out the prospect of understanding not only the hidden inner world, but also the mystifying outer world of power and powerlessness. It presumes the possibility of a postoedipal separation in which individuals are able to turn back and look at their parents, and to assess critically their legacy rather than simply identifying with their authority [which enables us to come to terms with difference].
>
> (Benjamin 1988: 180)

Benjamin, Chodorow (1989), Dimen and Goldner (2012), and Barden (2015) all demonstrate how a critical engagement with Oedipus, and moving beyond Oedipus, better fits the contemporary clinical scenarios we encounter. This is even more the case when working with trans persons (Lemma 2012, 2013). Yet, as therapists, the sheer complexity of working creatively with gender and sexuality, avoiding binary forms of splitting, is demanding, touching as they do on our own experiences, the ones we bring consciously and unconsciously to the intersubjective encounter. There is always something to recognise, something to learn, as we encounter the other in our clients and they encounter the other in us, redolent of past figures that appear so powerfully in the present, for good or ill. Saving the baby and throwing out the bathwater is demanding therapeutic work.

How do therapists work with evolving forms and expressions of gender and sexualities? Benjamin advocates the idea of the 'third' (2004, 2017). She argues that we best form our understanding of gender and sexuality through a 'mutually-created choreography that survives rupture . . . Rupture and repair could be described as a dyadic movement, an overarching process of the third that choreographs both partners. This movement creates new relational patterns or expectancies in both' (Benjamin 2013: 8). Or, to continue an overarching metaphor, a dancing landscape full of discovery, if we can take the risk of diverting from fixed paths. Self and other creates a 'thirdness' or a 'dance' that can rarely be created outside the consulting room, but that transmutes the past with the present to offer a new future based on mutual recognition involving rupture and repair. Gender is a core experience that forms our identity. Our challenge is to support clients as they engage with their external world, confronting issues of injustice or discrimination. The radical commitment of contemporary psychodynamic therapy, following in the footsteps of the radical nature of psychoanalysis in Freud's day, is to change the world on the inside and the outside in innovative ways, uniquely individual, embodied, inventive, sexual, and relational.

Focusing mainly on sexuality

Freud, who had profound things to say about sexuality, never had to deal with clients or patients traumatised by 'sexting'.

Anna's story

Anna cried, 'How could he do that to me? It was private. Now all his mates are having a laugh, staring at my tits'. Anna's distress was palpable as she, like many teenagers, had sent a revealing picture of herself via text to her boyfriend. After they split, his revenge was to send a picture to his 'mates'.

There are far too many stories of a young person who 'sexts' within the passion and intimacy of a relationship, only to discover their naked pictures being sent around to others and told 'it's just a bit of fun'. For Anna, it wasn't remotely funny, it was a form of abuse, and a further abuse of power that had led the relationship to end in the first place. It touched on gender, one of the four categories that make up our sexual identity, and how this gets distorted.

'Why do men think they can get away with everything? What gives them the right to control us women?'

Issues of our self-identity are inextricably entwined with our gender and our sexuality, however we identify ourselves. We continually receive 'messages' about who we are and how we 'should' be concerning sexuality from the media, friends, family, on-line communities, and other groups, all set within the framework of our society. The following clinical examples reveal how complex and multi-layered issues of gender and sexual identity are.

Angus's story

Angus was a young man who discovered he was homosexual in his teenage years. This posed a problem, as he was part of the school rugby team, which epitomised driven macho culture at a time when no well-known rugby players were 'out'. He hated the homophobic banter and eventually withdrew from the team, much to everyone's consternation, as he was one of the better players. He couldn't explain to the others why he had left, as it didn't feel safe, but he could not live a lie. Going to university gave Angus the freedom to try out his new identity.

Paul's story

I went to visit Paul in hospital. Despite being an old friend, we had lost touch. I was back in our home town so I decided to catch up, only to discover he had been taken into hospital with a life-threatening illness. I was given the name of the ward and, on navigating my way through the maze of the hospital, found myself standing outside a female surgical ward. Confused, I went in and saw Paul sitting up in bed, complete with a pink, frilly nightie – which sounds like a caricature but is completely true. Paul saw me, looked startled, even a little afraid, and then broke into a broad smile. He said, 'I bet you didn't expect this' and laughed, as did I. Paul had transitioned from a male to female identity several years earlier. He was living as a woman and was much happier with her new name, Pauline. Pauline told me counselling 'and a bit of surgery' had profoundly helped her. In fact, she had undergone two years of psychodynamic therapy, exploring her past and the links with her new identity. This had been a time of therapeutic transition, where she allowed herself to think of herself as a female in a male-gendered body. The containing and challenging experience offered by her therapist had made a huge difference to Pauline.

Gail's story

As a child, Gail's absolute favourite thing in life was to climb trees, no matter how high. In the park, her parents turned their backs for a few moments to arrange the family picnic, looked around, and couldn't see her. Gail shouted, 'I'm here', 30 feet up a tree, terrifying her parents. She was five years old.

Wind the clock forward 30 years and Gail is now a client. Gail's mother wanted her to be a girl just like her, interested in shopping, clothes, shoes, and handbags. Gail felt she had never been accepted, as none of these things ever appealed. At odds with her mother's vision, Gail longed for the outdoors. On holidays, she would pack a rucksack and go on walking and climbing adventures. Her photos showing her perched on some precarious rock-face still terrified her parents.

Gail had a profound sense of loss that she could not communicate with her mother, feeling an absence and a lack of affirmation that she was okay just as she was. Her mother had died the previous year with a rapidly spreading form of breast cancer. She was able to say to Gail in her last week of life, 'I do love you, you know', but Gail never felt it. She always felt her mother wanted her to be more of a stereotypical girl and less the adventurous tom-boy. Gail heard her mother's words but they did not touch her feelings.

Now Gail was working through a complicated form of grief, untangling her complex and ambivalent feelings.

Freud and sexuality

These brief stories take us into the heart of the complexities that exist around gender and sexual identity. Over a century earlier, Freud was concerned about sexuality and he, too, wanted to confront the sexual hypocrisy of his day. His earliest patients had been traumatised by sexual experiences, some actual and some Freud came to understand as originating in the mind of the patient. Freud evolved a new and shocking understanding of sexuality. His monumental work on dreams in 1900, and his *The Psychopathology of Everyday Life* (1901), captured people's imagination and became popular reading in the coffee-houses of Vienna. So he could not have done anything more calculated to offend people than by his

Three Essays on the Theory of Sexuality, published in 1905. This is Freud at his most controversial as he challenges the whole notion of sexuality as accepted at the turn of the last century. Before Freud, the understanding of sexuality was children do not have sexual feelings and childhood was a time-period before the emergence of sexual thoughts and feelings. The expectation was that women bear children and sexual intercourse was a duty. Sexual satisfaction (for men) was more likely to be found through a prostitute, mistress, or servant. It is estimated that in Freud's day, Vienna had 20,000 prostitutes (Tannahill 1980: 357), including children (with the age of consent being 14). These are captured in the images of a shocking Viennese artist of Freud's day, Egon Schiele (a protégée of Klimt), who drew many nude figures, including children. Schiele in turn influenced Tracy Emin, for whom sexuality is a central theme of her work as she, too, confronts contemporary attitudes towards sex.

Freud faced the hypocrisy of his time and context, with its denial, repression, and splitting, by developing a radically new idea about sexuality. He believed that a child's sexual life comes about spontaneously as an expression of who they are, although it later becomes focused on people, typically parents, represented through the Oedipus complex. A child's desire to discover and express sexuality comes from a very healthy instinct for knowledge.

Perversions and infantile sexuality

Freud's first essay (in *Three Essays*) was on sexual aberrations and dealt with the subject of perversions. Freud was confronting his readers with the extensive nature of sexuality, as it already existed – and from this evolved a theory that accounted for these as 'normal' expressions of sexuality. Freud therefore challenged the denial around sexuality, and enlarged our understanding of sexuality. Freud argued that what happened in adults had its origins in childhood. He then focused on infantile sexuality, expressing innate drives encountered through erogenous zones found in any part of the body that produces pleasurable feelings or excitement through use. This included either: the mouth – feeding, sucking, licking, biting; the anus – defecating, touching, contracting, penetration; the genitals – touching, masturbating; or the entire surface of the skin – holding, stroking, smelling, and so on. Freud compared these instinctual drives to interlinked canals, as different pleasures swap, change, and transform as the baby or child experiences, to use Freud's words, an unpleasure/pleasure principle at work. The mind avoids pain (unpleasure) and seeks pleasure, capturing the Freudian idea of polymorphously perverse sexuality. The baby doesn't care how it is pleasured, what it is pleasured with, or where it gets its pleasure from. Freud located the pleasure principle in the id and, as a baby develops psychologically, so does the ego, the location of the reality principle.

Freud saw all these actions and activities as adult foreplay that is a precursor to and prepares one for sexual intercourse. In this way, he balanced instinctual pleasure-seeking with the relational reality of adult life and evolutionary survival through procreation and sexual enjoyment. Yet this sexual desire, if repressed in a way that does not deny the essential being of the person, can also be transformed into a source of creativity. For Freud, sexuality was a dynamic presence or force that courses through us, seeking pleasure, avoiding inhibition and obstruction. It makes us alive and it pushes us to the abyss. It inflames and it engulfs. Sexual obsessions, like all obsessions, become compulsive, all-encompassing, and are not restrained by rational thought. These wild passions are played out in the unrestrained world of the psyche where we get some glimpses of our violence, obsessions, passions, and eroticism in the surrealism of our dreams. Yet the human race cannot survive on sexuality alone, no matter how much it craves.

Freud identified that we learn to balance the emergence of sexual identity and expression through processes of socialisation and enculturation. These wider social contexts give messages about what is acceptable and what is not, although these are often contested and change. One of the most important of these was the incest taboo that Freud located in the resolution of the Oedipal conflict. It was this taboo that Freud understood as a precursor to the origins of primitive belief systems. He believed that psychoanalysis was a more evolved belief system that did away with primitive beliefs such as dependence on a God, but in turn he did not reject the incest taboo. In *Civilization and Its Discontents* (1930), Freud argued there is a balance that individuals and societies need to strike. We need prohibitions and restrictions in order to determine what is good for the whole, not just for the individual, but it should not be assumed that these social norms are imposed unthinkingly or unfeelingly on each person. For example, as a doctor, Freud would have been committed to the sanctity of life as a principle held for the common good, yet Freud also chose to ask his personal doctor to end his long suffering and his life by an overdose of morphine.

As we saw earlier in the chapter, if the Oedipal understanding of gendered and sexual development needs revising, or replacing as Benjamin, Barden, and others argue, this calls into question how we live with no Oedipal restraint.

Sexuality in clinical practice

There are three ways in which psychodynamic therapists engage with sexuality and balancing the needs of the individual with the good of society.

First, there are multiple remnants or repeats of Freud's polymorphously perverse sexuality, some of which are approved of or disapproved of by the society in which we live, the norms of which change over time. There is always a struggle involved as we re-work these, in part because they are unconscious representations of our core sexuality. For example, one such remnant relates to oral satisfaction, as an unconscious desire to be fed, nurtured, and wanted. This includes smoking, eating, taking drugs, and consuming alcohol. Each of these activities becomes problematic when they are used to meet deeper psychological needs.

In our contemporary world, sexuality, sexual expression, and sexual orientations are, like gender, multi-layered. Sexuality touches every area of life, both in our clients and ourselves, so it is something that needs to be spoken about. Our sexuality and how we express it contributes to or detracts from the self we are now and are trying to become. This is an on-going balancing act with which many people struggle throughout life and is an important, but often overlooked, factor in many seeking therapy. It is almost as if we live in a world where sexuality has become common-place and we are looking for something else, something more intimate and deeper. It seems there is an even greater need for forms of attachment and experiences of trust, tenderness, and belonging, as well as our need to express our sexuality.

Second, an issue that Freud failed to address was power, in part because he occupied a male, intellectual, privileged elite that was blind to what they both possessed and used to oppress. While he acknowledged the dangers of power, hence his wolf analogy in *Civilization*, his solution was to focus on the need for some control at a societal level in order to avoid an even worse prospect of anarchy. However, while identifying the problem, his solution failed to see how power becomes expressed through language, gender, sexuality, and oppressive structures within society. It can also become oppressive by psychoanalytic systems when a client's experience of their sexual orientation is pathologised by the imposition of the therapist's theoretical understanding or experience in analysis (Friedman 2009). Any form of contemporary psychodynamic therapy needs to engage with the client's inner world in the context of their outer world. It also explains the reason why relational psychoanalysis, Lacanian analysis, and contemporary forms of therapy need to begin with the power dynamic present in the therapy room, expressed through the language we use and how this shapes the intersubjective encounter. Therapists always need to be attentive to issues of power as it influences us in subtle ways beyond the immediately apparent. Clients will challenge our unspoken norms and, in responding well, we have the opportunity to enter into an authentic intersubjectivity – one that is conducive to a mutual revealing of the unconscious. Yet the challenge to our power can elicit a defensiveness that results in *inauthentic* intersubjectivity, especially in the areas of gender and sexuality. Students and supervisees still tell me of stories of their encounters with therapists that I would view as shockingly homophobic and often repeats early patterns. While some of this may be theoretical (Friedman 2009), Sandler (2009) takes the view that it can be because of a failure in clinical technique when working with the counter-transference. (We shall return to how we work with counter-transference in Chapter 13.)

Third, we need to be alive to the presence of sexuality and the power of fantasy in the therapy room. Psychodynamic therapy is a psychologically intimate experience. Our clients tell us things they have rarely or never shared with another person.

Esther's story

Esther said, 'We then went to have sex in the woods'.

I was surprised, as Esther and Jerry's relationship had hit an all-time low, making this a very unexpected development. There was another problem. I suffer from tinnitus in my left ear, so often all I can hear is a high-pitched whistle. This means I can mishear what people say.

I asked Esther, 'Sex in the woods, is that something you normally do?' She burst out laughing. 'No', she said. 'Jerry wanted to cook eggs in the woods. Sex was the last thing on my agenda'. I thought cooking eggs in the woods was far stranger than having sex there.

When the fixed number of counselling sessions came to an end (I was being paid by her employer), we agreed to continue on an open-ended basis. While my physical hearing was impaired on this occasion, it transpired my unconscious hearing was attuned to the issue Esther really wanted to talk about. She explained that, until she had the security of knowing that the therapy could be on-going (rather than a limited number of sessions) and that I wanted to work with her, she couldn't feel brave enough to talk about her grooming and abuse by a family friend she had trusted. Esther was confused about her sexuality, power and powerlessness, and what kind of woman she wanted to be.

Esther's story, in principle though not in the details, is a common one. Clients are searching not just for meaning, but for an identity, one that is gendered and sexual.

Summary

Esther reminds us that sex, fantasy, gender identity, and power are always in the counselling or therapy room and need to be addressed. This is even more so when working with adolescents (Luxmore 2016), who always have something to teach us. Yet therapists, too, need to attend to their own sexuality. The intimacy of the therapeutic encounter can be as powerful as any physical intimacy. Clients do fall in love with their therapists, often becoming dependent. The therapists I supervise view their greatest clinical struggles as cases where they did not identify the power of erotic transference early in the work (see Chapter 13). It can lead to the therapy ending abruptly, which is neither helpful for the client nor the therapist. Nothing unethical has happened, but the therapist feels they have let their client down. It is when therapists ignore the presence of the power of sex, the erotic, fantasy, and sexuality in the counselling room, that they can slip into stereotypical patterns related to male power, desire, and domination. These set the scene for boundary violations (Gabbard 2016) that litter the history of psychoanalysis, psychotherapy, and counselling (all modalities), although these professions are by no means unique in this regard.

This raises the wider issues of how and why things go wrong for people, ourselves included, in the early years of life. Unsurprisingly, many traumas revolve around the failure or absence of bonds of love, as well as the abuse of power, often related to gender and sexual identity. These and other factors underpin a psychodynamic understanding of psychopathology that forms the subject of the next chapter.

Reflective questions

How do you feel about your gendered body and identity?

Should you raise this as an issue with your current or future clients? If not, why not?

What are the most challenging aspects of gender or sexualities for psychodynamic practice?

Looking at research

Some chapters focusing on research are found in Fonagy, Leuzinger-Bohleber, and Krause's (2009) edited book, *Identity, Gender and Sexuality: 150 Years After Freud*.

The British Psychoanalytic Council has published a bibliography of key publications, including some focusing on research (primarily qualitative). Available at: https://www.bpc.org.uk/sites/psychoanalytic-council.org/files/BPC%20Bibliography%20%28Sexual%20Orientations%29.pdf [accessed 17 July 2018].

PART 4
Clinical Perspectives

12

When life goes wrong – introducing psychopathology and trauma

What is unique about trauma is that it is unique to each person. Everybody experiences trauma in some form or another. It has been an inescapable part of life for as long as the human race has existed. So step back in time and imagine being a Roman legionnaire defending Hadrian's Wall from marauding Scots. Well-organised and well-armed legionnaires decimated their opponents, leaving many dead or lying bleeding on the ground, traumatised – literally – as trauma is the Greek word for 'wound'. This word, 'trauma', has passed into our language to describe physical and psychological experiences where some aspect of us has been pierced, penetrated, or damaged: physically, having fallen down a mountain, I was being treated for multiple traumas to my body, being told by a hospital consultant 'with time you will heal'; psychologically, I experienced helplessness, abandonment, anger – 'Why is this happening to me?' – with some flashbacks as if replaying in slow motion every millisecond of my fall (Ross 2014, 2016a).

As you read this, if it triggers memories of your own traumas, I am sorry if that causes you regret or pain, even now often years after the event. From a psychodynamic perspective, trauma is what goes on in the mind as well as the body. Trauma is the consequence of a sudden and overwhelming event that leaves us unprepared to face it, and that overwhelms our normal patterns of coping or making sense of things. This event can be external, internal, or both. The consequence of trauma can be a profound impact on our psychological functioning with short- and long-term consequences.

Psychical trauma refers to an event in a person's life that has an emotional, violent, or shocking intensity that shakes the foundations, or opens up a wound, in the psyche. Over time, this affects the whole structure of the psyche and its operation, expressed in forms of psychopathology. In this chapter, we shall see why psychodynamic therapy offers a different vision of psychopathology and how people make sense of their distress when life falls apart or threatens to do so. Psychopathology, understood from a dynamic perspective, pays attention to what goes on in the psyche, the unique mind of each person. It is distinct from psychiatric diagnosis that purports to apply to entire populations based on deviations from 'normal' thoughts, feelings, and behaviours (Davey 2014). It shifts the emphasis from 'What is wrong with you?' to 'What has happened to you?' Yet, much psychopathology has its origins in some form of trauma, especially sexual trauma in the form of abuse. Trauma is one side of the coin, recovery is the other (Herman 1992) – an essential task that is part of the Freudian DNA of dynamic therapies.

Freud and trauma

Psychoanalysis came into being because Freud was willing to take seriously the trauma of his early women patients. Herman describes and critiques the origins of trauma in Freud. Breuer first spoke about following the thread of memory from the present into the past and Freud took this up in his case histories. These reveal his curiosity, his willingness to explore areas of sexuality in his patients as they told him stories of sexual assault, exploitation, abuse, and incest. In a report of 18 case studies, entitled *The Aetiology of Hysteria*, he made a dramatic claim:

> I therefore put forward the thesis that at the bottom of every case of hysteria there are *one or more occurrences of premature sexual experience*, occurrences which belong to the earliest years of childhood ... A century later this paper still rivals contemporary clinical descriptions of the effects of childhood sexual abuse. It is a brilliant, compassion, eloquently argued [document].
>
> (Herman 1992: 130)

Yet within two years, Freud rejected this 'seduction hypothesis' because of an awareness of the profound social and cultural implications. As a physician working in private practice in Vienna, to advance such ideas could lead to academic ridicule, social isolation, failure, and poverty, Freud's worst fears (Ross 2016b). The paradox is this led to his focus on the workings of the psyche, including unconscious processes involving the sexual drive, fantasy, and repression – the building blocks of the early psychoanalysis and how we understand psychopathology.

Starting with psychopathology

Each of us has our own experience of psychopathology and our own unique psychopathology linked to our personal story.

I wandered down the grim, dank hallways of an immense Victorian building, Claybury Psychiatric Hospital (now closed). In the corridors, I would meet patients, nurses, and doctors where some would gaze fixedly ahead, oblivious to the world around. Others would nod curtly, and then continue on a path they alone knew. I was on my way to run a therapy group on an acute admission unit. Here, I was often left with the question, 'Why?' Why do some people get ill and some people do not, even if what on the surface seems a similar event? 'On the surface' implies there is so much that goes on below the surface of which we are barely conscious. Even taking into account the genetic predispositions for some mental illnesses; addictive behaviours, such as alcoholism; and destructive or risk behaviours – why do some people get depressed? What triggers the depth of despair? Why does anxiety overwhelm and paralyse? How is it that abuse is experienced as lifelong trauma by some people, while others survive without burying such awful events? A need to explain 'why' lies behind the need for psychiatric diagnosis and psychopathology, not just in psychiatry but in psychology, counselling, and psychotherapy as well. Unless we understand how something, or more likely *someone*, goes wrong, we have less chance of being able to find a solution, alleviate the symptoms, or offer any form of hope or healing, relational or otherwise.

Writing on psychopathology follows a common pattern: a definition of what constitutes a mental disorder; a list of signs and symptoms found in specific mental disorders (that indicate their pathology); concluding with what treatments are available and their relative effectiveness (Castonguay and Oltmanns 2013; Davey 2014). Psychopathology has become dominated by the Diagnostic and Statistical Manual of Mental Disorders (DSM), now in its fifth edition (APA 2013). Controversial as this has become for medicalising mental illness and the influence of pharmaceutical firms (Davies 2014), its limitations have been addressed by the much more holistic and independent Psychodynamic Diagnostic Manual (PDM), now in its second edition (Lingiardi and McWilliams 2017).

Psychodynamic psychopathology takes a different focus by looking at the unique impact on the individual and the personal meaning they make of the symptoms they are encountering. Contemporary psychodynamic therapists want to examine why this particular event was felt in that particular way. What sense did they make of it, rationally and emotionally? Clients tell us of their greatest pleasures and greatest pain or traumas. We enter into the agonies and ecstasies of extraordinary lives found in the ordinariness of living. We help clients explore why they repeat actions that cause them angst. We bear their anger and rage at being powerless, as we too become powerless in the grip of their re-enacted story, contained safely within the walls of the counselling room. We explore their unfulfilled, aching longings. In and through these explorations in therapy, a person can discover unconscious aspects of themselves, and with insight make different choices for the future.

Implicit in our basic assumptions are the notions of what life can be like if all goes well, emerging out of relationships where we encounter bonds of love, forming a healthy psyche and sense of self. The hallmark of such a self is the conviction without illusion that 'I am loved and wanted in this world'. From such a foundation, anything is possible. It is important as therapists that we do not lose sight of this visionary potential as a way of seeing the other. Given that psychoanalysis had its origins in observing the traumas of Freud and Breuer's early patients (1893–1895), the focus is more often on what happens when there is a lack, a failure, a delay, or something or someone is missing at a crucial time when a person develops their unique mind, psyche, and sense of self. At its simplest, dynamic forms of psychopathology all involve early trauma, often pre-verbal, that can: stretch back through the generations (Alpert 2015); emerge from conception and be present in utero (Weinstein 2016); be experienced at birth (Winnicott 1949) and repeated in and through early bonding or through the failure to bond, leading to later forms and expressions of embodied trauma (Lemma 2010); compromise neural patterns (Solomon and Siegel 2003); disrupt attachments (Fonagy 2001); or lead to traumatic attachments that resist adaptation and change (Brothers 2014).

Breaking through

What is significant is when trauma or traumas break through what Freud thought of as a protective shield (1920), although it was later analysts, such as Winnicott and Khan, that saw this protective role as the function of the mother, and of particular importance in cumulative trauma (Khan 1963). The question of early trauma and the idea of a 'basic fault' were first developed by Michael Balint, a Hungarian psychoanalyst who worked with Ferenczi, one of Freud's early colleagues (Szekacs-Weisz and Keve 2012a, 2012b). The power of the unconscious is such that trauma can remain dormant but not extinct, like a volcano able to erupt at any time. When it does erupt, when the trauma breaks through, Balint sees this as the formation of a 'basic fault' (Balint 1968; Stewart 1996). One understanding of Balint's basic fault is that it is formed by early trauma caused by a mismatch between the needs of the person and the failure of the people who form the external environment (Balint 1958, 1968).

In any subsequent trauma, the client regresses to the pattern of the original basic fault and replicates or regresses to the type of object relation present at that time. This becomes a trauma-located fault-line capable of future movements in the shifting psyche. Balint locates the timing of a basic fault before the splitting of Klein, which forms another defensive structure to enable the emerging infant's self to survive attacks, internal or external, often experienced as traumatic.

Real events impinge on the protective structures of the psyche and, as a consequence, these damage or disrupt psychic structures and attack the emerging sense of self (Balint 1969). This can have a much more traumatic impact when such protective structures are still being formed or less well-developed, and Freud believed it was such trauma-related events that would respond well to analysis (1937). Freud also believed that trauma becomes a part of us in our internal world and reappears through dreams that link the person back to the time and place of the original trauma. A key example of this was Freud's case study of 'Little Hans' (1909), the analysis of Herbert Graf by his father, Max Graf. Freud saw Hans once and supervised his father from 1906 to 1908. The case concerned Hans' precocious sexuality and obsession with penises ('widdlers'). Found masturbating, his mother threatened to cut it off, and Hans subsequently had anxiety-filled dreams of a horse biting him, where horses were to be feared because they had big widdlers. The dream was triggered by the trauma of the arrival of a sister when he was three-and-a-half and was understood in conventional Oedipal terms. The originating trauma and his repressed aggression at being displaced led to his anxiety. Hans ultimately lost his fear of horses and his general anxiety and developed a good relationship with his father. He visited Freud in 1922 but had little recollection of these early events.

Trauma and splitting

Splitting is the process where we separate positive feelings about ourselves or others from negative feelings so that we, or they, are experienced as all good or all bad. The capacity to split can become a division in the psyche and becomes built into how the person experiences relationships and engages with the external world. Psychopathology reveals other splits between: language and meaning; fantasy and reality; thinking and feeling; deadness and aliveness; or expression and denial. These splits are commonly experienced in and through the relationship in the counselling room.

Many of these splits can be observed in the emotional backdrop of the intertwined histories of many fractured and tormented lives trapped in the past at the hands of others. We, like our clients, may have less dramatic but equally fractured lives. Such fractures may be expressed in the categories used in conventional psychopathology: depression; generalised anxiety disorder; panic disorder and phobias; obsessive-compulsive disorder; post-traumatic stress disorder (PTSD); eating disorders; substance use disorders; personality disorders; bipolar disorder; and marital and relational discord (Castonguay and Oltmanns 2013). Behind these categories lie deeper splits in the psyche that become exposed.

While some of these may feature and be a factor in our distress, clients come with a malaise of the soul, existential angst, despair and depression, feelings of imminent breakdown and an irrevocable falling apart, a splintering or fracturing of the psyche, a barely contained cap on volcanic anger or molten rage, unmourned ghosts that still haunt, often allied to guilt (real or imagined) and irreducible feelings of shame. Yet, despite such catastrophic feelings, there remains throughout a constant but faint echo of a yearning for redemption, a wistful longing for a home, and a flickering candle of hope even through the storms of the psyche.

Clients come to therapy searching for something so that, by re-visiting the past, somehow things might be different for the present and the future. An obvious place to start is by listening to the rehearsed narrative, but also to the unspoken narrative that emerges in the room, in our thinking and feelings, and in the gaps. As contemporary psychodynamic and integrative therapists, we are interested in discovering a person's story and piecing together what might have been, and what serves as an unlocking metaphor for their narrative. Invariably, there are many traumas hidden within each client and these need to be explored to locate a person within their narrative, within their psyche, and the meaning of events and other people. What we are looking for is not any old trauma, but those traumas, individual or cumulative, that have or have the potential to become toxic if not attended to.

Adapting to the client's case

It is vital to consider carefully the therapeutic skills that you utilise, adapting these to the needs of your client. Consider combat veterans. What we have learnt from US veterans of the Vietnam War (1965–1973), and soldiers from subsequent conflicts, is that talking therapies do not help everyone all of the time. While psychodynamic therapies are invaluable for psychic-based trauma (Mollon 1996), they do not address embodied trauma, or the range of symptoms now recognised as PTSD, to the same degree. New non-dynamic developments include Shapiro's (2001) eye movement desensitisation and reprocessing (EMDR), which offers a technique that has shown positive results. Mindfulness has its origins in Kabat-Zinn's cognitive-based engagement with combat veterans, and subsequently with those experiencing long-standing depression (Williams et al. 2007). Energy-based therapies, utilising the idea of innate energy systems in the body and the mind, have been applied to psychodynamic practice by Mollon (2004, 2008) with great effect. Leighton (2007) sees value in integrating many aspects of EMDR into intersubjective therapy, whilst acknowledging that some aspects are troubling when they detract from the relationship between client and therapist. Just as with psychodynamic therapies, a distinct but different kind of relatedness is necessary for each client.

There are times when a trauma can be treated using one of these methods. After the traumatic experience of my fall, where a great deal of the physical trauma was still embodied, I worked with a therapist who used a form of energy therapy called advanced integrative therapy (AIT) alongside her psychodynamic listening to and for the unconscious, to good effect. It identified a deeper, long-standing trauma that earlier therapy had identified but not addressed.

Sources of psychic trauma

Psychic trauma has three main sources, and it is entirely possible to encounter all three in one client, which greatly complicates the therapeutic task.

The first source of trauma comes from factors beyond any individual's control and is seen most clearly in: social and cultural repression (Herman 1992); inter-generational trauma (Rucker and Mermelstein 1979); the emotional casualties of endemic conflicts around the world (not all of which get into the news); being a refugee as a 'stranger in a strange land' with multiples losses at many levels (given the vast increase in the number of refugees,

Eleftheriadou [2016] sees an urgent need to create safe spaces offering psychotherapeutic support for refugees and provides insightful clinical examples); the experience of being a persecuted minority due to some form of 'difference' or 'otherness'; or, some difficult to define threat to the archetypal soul of a person in the collective or mythical unconscious (Kalsched 2013). This list is indicative only, as many other forms of trauma exist that precede a person's existence and reside in wider familial, social, and cultural forms.

Maya's story

Maya arrived in the UK as a refugee and was granted leave to remain. Her country was at civil war and so unsafe for her to return. Her village had been destroyed and its people had fled, scattered across the country and beyond its borders.

Maya wanted to train as a counsellor, having experienced great help from a psychiatrist and psychotherapist attached to Médecins Sans Frontières (Doctors Without Borders). She obtained a foundation qualification and was attending an introductory counselling skills course in preparation for accredited counsellor training. In one training session, she told her moving life-story but expressed no feelings. While fleeing, she was caught by a soldier and in order to protect her child, was brutally raped. Waiting until he was drunk and despite being wounded and bleeding, she escaped. As I looked around the group, they were in shock, as they felt the previously untold trauma of Maya. She was blasé saying, 'Oh that happened to everyone' and implied this was nothing new as it had been going on for decades. It was simply accepted as part of her culture, like much inter-generational trauma.

Maya did well on the course, with great empathic skills for others but less for herself. I suggested that she needed to process her trauma and suggested a therapist who had worked in other cultures. Maya saw a colleague that had worked with refugees in Africa and this created an immediate bond and an unspoken relationship was formed. Much of Maya's trauma came out in disturbing dreams that her psychodynamic therapist patiently listened to and helped Maya understand in culturally relevant ways. Maya also came to see how much trauma there had been in her early family that she took for granted as 'the way life was'. Now she was in another culture, she was also able to see the impact of belonging to a persecuted tribe on the fringe of her society. Much of her trauma was embodied and her therapist helped her connect with these split-off parts of her body.

Several years later, Maya sent me a picture of her graduation, with a beaming smile and big, brown eyes no longer haunted. My hope is that Maya's experience of inter-generational trauma may have been contained, at least in part, for her daughter's sake.

Another aspect of trauma is, of course, our own life experience in the womb, at birth and beyond. Much is inaccessible to us but retained within unconscious psychic memory, and so capable of being triggered by events, such as the birth of our own child. It comes as a shock to some parents that seeing their baby thrive triggers old wounds from their own childhood. A parent can come to envy the care their own baby receives. This can cause tensions between partners, with one believing the baby is getting more attention than they are. They feel left out, abandoned, isolated. Hurt, this re-awakens unconscious patterns (that are often repeats from before) marked by: being emotionally absent; being overly controlling; projecting bad feelings into the baby or the mother; feeling excessively anxious or depressed; experiencing intrusive thoughts that somehow everything is their fault; and with the malaise of some kind of unspoken doom awaiting. In the worst cases there can also be violence against the baby or the mother.

Being attentive to our past, and its various traumas, is a key aspect of our own work in personal therapy because it prepares us to be able to work with others at the depth they require if early childhood material is triggered.

The second source of trauma covers areas that examine the provision of healthy developmental processes, good attachments, the formation of an interpersonal self, vital mother–baby interactions, and the creation of healthy neural pathways (touched on in Chapters 8–10). The absence of these can cause trauma and include: physical health difficulties in the baby or the mother; psychological or mental health issues impinging on this vital relationship; nurturing or bonding issues; as well as family dysfunction, social problems, and financial difficulties (Raphael-Leff 2015; Acquarone 2016). These various factors get played out and expressed through absence, failure, neglect, and insecure or ambivalent attachments, all situated in and around early interpersonal relationships (Beebe and Lachmann 2002; Renn 2012). Further trauma-related factors include: difficulty in conceiving and the traumas of in vitro fertilisation; a history of multiple miscarriages and the consequent mingled and confused hopes and fears; being a 'replacement' baby for one that died, often with the same name; being fostered or adopted, leaving a gap in knowledge and feelings with no one to ask; being an unplanned or, more damagingly, an unwanted pregnancy; premature birth and life in a neo-natal ward; a long and difficult labour; and an inability to bond or connect with the newborn infant leading to overwhelming guilt, as well as feelings of failure (Weinstein 2016).

In working with clients, it is always helpful to get a full a picture of what they know or have been told about their origins. What I have learnt about myself includes: being an unplanned pregnancy; financial hardship causing a lack of a healthful diet for my mother; a sudden unexpected birth, two months premature; no one knowing it was a twin pregnancy so, in the words of the nurse, 'Oh look there's another one', me; weighing 3 lbs (Liz) and 4 lbs (me), respectively; being fed milk hourly via a tête de pipette; spending our first nights together in a shoe box (in a cot) – bizarre as that sounds, it was confirmed by my grandmother; wearing dolls' clothes that had been knitted overnight; and being described as looking like 'skinned rabbits'. As our birth weights dropped, Liz hit her target weight of six pounds and left the maternity unit after three weeks. It took me longer and I went home after five weeks. As a consequence in adult life, I have learnt to survive, and there is a driven part of me that will ensure that happens. When my climbing accident could have been life-threatening (Ross 2014, 2016a), my psyche revealed a steely determination and, as a psychoanalyst colleague said, 'your capacity to go into your mind and not be overwhelmed by multiple injuries helped you survive'. At other times, I note I can be ruthless and I attribute this to some sense of unconscious threat that gets activated.

Recalling these events as a therapist tells me several things. First, normal life is full of healthy attachments and the pain of separations, yet I often find it difficult to end with clients as I become attached to them, and they to me. My traumatic separation from my twin in the first weeks of life may make separation a greater issue for me now as a therapist.

Even without any experience of traumatic separation, the task of separation (and identity) is a lifelong issue for twins (Lewin 2004). Second, it is important to work with the 'basic fault' and not be diverted by simply focusing on the specific presenting trauma, complex and painful as that may be. Third, whatever traumas are encountered, they can be overcome, and I am in awe of the bravery of so many clients, especially when they have experienced toxic levels of trauma. Fourth, being present with clients in reliable, containing ways, whether short- or long-term, that sees their basic fault, identifies their fractured psyche, and holds their splits are all expressions of bonds of love. I am using Benjamin's phrase in a wider, metaphorical sense than her focus on gender, sexuality, and power. Fraiberg and colleagues express this with the metaphor of ghosts:

> In every nursery there are ghosts. They are the visitors from the unremembered past of the parents, the uninvited guests at the christening. Under favorable circumstances, these unfriendly and unbidden spirits are banished from the nursery and return to their subterranean dwelling place. The baby makes his own imperative claim upon parental love and, in strict analogy with the fairy tales, the *bonds of love* protect the child and his parents against the intruders, the malevolent ghosts.
>
> (Fraiberg, Adelson, and Shapiro quoted in Kalsched 2003: 152; italics added)

Toxic trauma

Malevolent ghosts are a fitting analogy for the third source of trauma, the toxic effect of a person's deliberate harm of another through an abuse of power expressed in physical, sexual, spiritual, or psychological forms. Toxin in the psyche can kill, if not the body, then the soul.

I was climbing up a narrow path through a forested area en route to the plateau region of Mount Mulanje in Malawi. I had just passed a rocky area when suddenly Jack (my son-in-law) shouted out in alarm. I turned to see him looking pale as a large brownish-green snake slithered away into the undergrowth. From the markings, we later identified it as a female Boomslang, a snake whose venomous bite can be fatal. In my experience, the effect of some people on others are just as toxic, just as deadly as if bitten by a poisonous snake. Sadly, listening to the awful histories of clients can reveal, all too powerfully, the truth about how poisonous some people are to their children.

A sad indictment of our humanity is our capacity to exploit one another, especially those who are vulnerable and powerless, imprinting the most toxic traumas. Thirty years ago, my wife was an administrator for Social Services and used to take minutes for the Child Abuse Register. I, like she, was shocked to discover that many of the people on the list included solicitors, doctors, teachers, and other professionals. Our naïve understanding of abuse at that time, blinded by class and privilege, was that sexual abuse happened, but not in nice middle-class suburbs and amongst educated professionals.

Gary and Tom's stories

A friend Gary told me about his experience of sexual exploitation while at boarding school. Aged only eight, he felt this was just part of his overwhelming unhappiness at that time. He mentioned this when we were playing darts at a local pub in an offhand, casual manner. He felt he had been far more deeply influenced by the death of a friend and told me he didn't need therapy. On the surface I agreed with him, wondering what was going on in his unconscious.

Another friend, Tom, also trapped in a boarding school context, experienced what would now be seen as a paedophile ring and suffered frequent abuse. His parents worked abroad. This school had a prestigious name and academic reputation but it destroyed his sense of self. Tom struggled academically though eventually found a career he loved. He also met a woman he loved but found it difficult to be sexually alive. I suggested Tom seek therapy. Trusting was enormously difficult, yet in therapy he came to realise that he had developed dissociative identity disorder (DID) and found a suitable therapist with experience in this area.

What is dissociative identity disorder?

The toxic nature of trauma can result in DID (formerly known as multiple personality), which used to be regarded as a rare psychological problem. We have now come to realise it is a common response to early and severe – often sexual – abuse, one that enables the person to survive at the time but at great cost. It describes the separation of mental states within the person, unbeknownst to them, that helps them to maintain two ways of being where they are not aware there is any contradiction.

As we saw in Chapter 5, repression plays a vital part of psychodynamic identity. It has a positive role to play in protecting the psyche from being overwhelmed. The problem is that repression does not accommodate dissociation of the mind into multiple states of consciousness contained in the unconscious. The last twenty years has seen a growth in research, understanding, and clinical encounters related to the emergence of disassociation (Sinason 2002, 2012). At its most extreme, the person may exist through several independent personalities, each unaware of the other. A colleague has done very creative work with her DID client where she gets one 'person', say the abandoned six-year-old, to help another 'person', say the abused two-year-old, to cope, whilst both of them remain unaware of a third 'person', for instance a very angry teenager who appears whenever there is any threat or change. This therapist has enabled all three personalities to work together where the six-year-old no longer feels abandoned, the two-year-old feels safe now somebody else knows, and the teenager can understand why she is so angry. Having a friend with DID was very different but began to make sense of some of the curious absences that marked our friendship. If we think about it, every one of us is in touch with someone who has experienced some form of abuse. So why was it that Gary seemed okay and Tom was very troubled? Knowing Tom much better, I knew about his early life, the lack of boundaries in his family, the emotional volatility of his father, and the crushing presence of his mother who took an inappropriate interest in his cleanliness when bathing him. She took little interest in the rest of his life and all his early years he was brought up by a nanny until the departure for boarding school. Tom came to see he did not trust women, sought male company, and found himself in ambivalent relationships. His basic fault could be an absence of intimacy but with an unfulfilled longing for it. Looking back, Tom felt he became vulnerable to exploitation in his later life.

Contemporary psychodynamic thinking, incorporating new knowledge of trauma drawn from neuroscience, multiple self-states, multiple intersubjectivities, and the potential for the co-creation of relationships, is able to address the complex issues raised by disassociation (Howell and Itzkowitz 2016). In order to avoid overwhelming trauma, such repression is required that it leads to either a split in the psyche or the formation of another enclaved part of the psyche expressed as other forms of consciousness. As Mollon illustrates,

> I once asked a patient with DID how she created a new personality. She replied . . . 'when something bad is happening, I withdrew further and further from it – until there is just a space where I used to be – and in that space a new personality forms'.
>
> (2012: 19)

Dissociation comes about as a psychological consequence of trauma, ritualistic forms of abuse, torture, and war, but the most common cause comes through extreme or repeated sexual abuse at a very early pre-verbal stage of development. While all psychodynamic therapists need to be aware of the possibility that early trauma can cause dissociative states in their clients, working with clients who have more developed patterns of DID is challenging and requires specialist supervision – and possibly further training. In working with dissociative clients, the key skill is to identify and work with the main aspect of the person, while addressing the needs of the earlier parts of the client that have been overlooked and are often very angry. Another way of working with such clients is to pay careful attention to somatisation and identify the trauma located in the body of the person. Why such early trauma is so damaging to the psyche needs further exploration.

Impact of sexual trauma

Historically, psychoanalysis has had difficulties in addressing sexual trauma. While Freud never gave up his early 'seduction hypothesis', the idea that the sexual abuse of his early patients resulted in their later hysterical and obsessional traumas, he focused more on the power of sexuality, fantasy, and desire as part of the development of the psyche, as expressed in the Oedipus complex. He elaborated processes in the mind rather than encounters in the body. Later psychoanalytic thinkers, such as Laplanche (1987), have developed more complex understandings of sexuality, which offer new insights into the psychodynamic impact of abuse. As contemporary psychodynamic therapy examines both, holding together the inner and outer worlds of the client, much more is now understood about the complex traumas to the self, psyche, mind, and soul brought about by sexual abuse.

An attack at the core of the psyche

Laplanche developed a distinctive understanding of the unconscious, which contributes to our understanding of trauma. He separates the unconscious into repressed and enclaved parts. The enclaved unconscious is encapsulated where no psychic thinking or symbolic representation takes place. When an adult sexually abuses a child, this stems from an enclaved unconscious that inserts something into the child's psyche that cannot be thought about, translated, or symbolised, a form of enigmatic message. The violent process of intromission ruptures the child's development, as the abuse locates something unrepresentable or untranslatable in the child's psyche. Stein adds,

> Trauma in a Laplanchian framework is an uninterpretable intromission of untranslatable messages that deteriorate into sinister, garbled, 'untranslatable' missives of the superego: it is characterized by messages that emerge from some psychotic persecutory enclave.
>
> (2007: 188).

As therapists, we work with sexually abused clients whose core psyche has been attacked, resulting in 'occupying' and destructive objects that seek opportunity to come to life, just like hungering, devouring ghosts, as well as a critical, persecutory super-ego or aspects of the self.

A distortion of the bonds of love and the proliferation of shame

How can a child make sense of the powerful switch from a sense of being wanted to an experience of being used? It is as if individual feelings and affections no longer matter. It creates the idea that as a person I exist for the needs of others and come alive only when others want me or need me, not that I exist for myself. Abuse survivors record how they learnt to view relationships in sexualised terms and how destructive this was in the formation of their sexual identity.

Shame as a tool of abuse

Sadly, there is another dimension of shame occurring through sexual abuse. A key driver in further psychological trauma, in addition to sexual trauma, is the deliberate use of shame as a tool to manipulate or control by the abuser. This is especially felt by those who have experienced grooming, the purposeful and insidiously destructive exploitation of another over a sustained period of time, often years, playing on vulnerability and manipulating trust. Shame appears to be endemic and like a virulent, health-threatening superbug, resistant to existing antibiotics or psychodynamic therapy. In part, this is because of the lack of recognition of the shame the therapist brings into the room with their client. Shame is not always a client issue. Orange believes that any shame found in the consulting room does not belong to the client or the therapist because it is 'intersubjectively generated, maintained, exacerbated, and, we hope, mitigated within the relational system . . . No one is born ashamed, but, paralyzed, we can surely inhabit together experiential worlds' (2008: 85).

Sally's story

Sally started therapy because of problems of intimacy and stated, 'I'm very good at sex, you know. I like sex, but I can't be doing with all that lovey-dovey nonsense'. She said this with a smile on her face, as if looking for a reaction. I felt she was trying to shock me and take control of the new situation she was uncomfortable with. At some stage in the session I said something like, 'I feel you are trying to shock because I think something shocking has happened to you in the past, something that fills you with so much shame you always need to be in control'. Sally looked shocked and, although she was not audibly crying, tears began to trickle down her face.

My interpretation of her words drawn from my counter-transferential feelings caught her hidden shame. It emerged Sally was terrified of intimacy and, in our two years working together, we were to discover why when a history of abuse emerged alongside profound feelings of shame. Her abuser had always made her feel it was her fault. Sally felt she had a shameful secret she could never tell, but now she could.

Unconscious coercion or manipulation as a 'normal' part of a relational dynamics

The experience of being abused can have devastating consequences for the person, and for their future, as what is thought to be 'normal' becomes distorted.

Kari's story

Kari's violent, drunken father sexually abused him and there was a sense of relief when he left the family home for prison. Kari later sexually abused his youngest sister. He was doing what had been done to him, but later in therapy found it extraordinarily difficult to cope with the knowledge he was both a victim and a perpetrator.

'I hate myself. Even now in every relationship at work, with friends or family, an instinctive part of me is looking how I can get what I want'.

Kari's ambivalence was around the fact he was a very successful car salesman (that made a bonus every month). He was concerned that if he changed, he might lose his career. Therapy enabled Kari to discover uncomfortable truths about himself, but this was also a very demanding piece of clinical work that required a thoughtful, careful balancing act to avoid stigmatising and shaming him. Clinical supervision was especially helpful in enabling me to see what unconscious, punitive dynamics were being worked out, potentially repeating earlier abusive processes. I, too, could become the abuser in an apparently therapeutic role if I got caught up in Kari's ambivalence and failed to see him as a victim.

The negative impact on attachment patterns and family systems

We saw in Chapter 9 how important attachment patterns are for healthy psychological development. Abuse attacks these attachments and distorts them.

Jill's story

Jill had a love/hate relationship with her sister. She always felt plain, 'frumpy', never the 'life and soul' of the party like her sister, Janice. Later, the family discovered her father and uncle had abused Janice. At one level, the family 'knew', but something was never spoken and nobody put all the clues together. Jill was very angry with her mother for not protecting Janice and for neglecting her. In one session, bristling with anger, Jill shouted, 'At least if I had been abused I would have got some attention!'

She had learnt to keep herself safe by becoming invisible. However now, in her mid-thirties, she was estranged from her sister, 'still acting the drama queen', resented being overlooked at work, taken for granted by her ill mother, and felt unloved by her partner.

Jill and Janice had both been 'abused' as part of the systemic nature of the family. Both developed complex attachment patterns that they replicated throughout life. Therapists can so focus on the past abuse they fail to see the on-going impact of abuse expressed in on-going powerlessness misinterpreted as resistance or being stuck. The fear of being seen evokes feelings of stigma and betrayal, in the wider family context and in the therapy room. They long for the truth to be told and to engage in authentic dialogue but so often hide camouflaged by their guilt, shame, and blame of themselves.

Instilling helplessness, rage, and betrayal

What does it feel like to be helpless or powerless when any vestige of control is taken away? I recall a memory of being beaten up by a gang as a teenager. It was nothing serious, a black eye and a bruised ego, but it left its mark. For most of my teenage years, I dreamt of revenge, discovering a depth of anger in me, an emotion I was unfamiliar with. Yet this pales by comparison with the rage I see in abused clients. It emerges when clients recall events or memories, often fragmentary, but emerging unexpectedly with a visceral power that feels like a shock-wave in the counselling room. Often that rage is focused on the act of betrayal. In betrayal, someone we depended upon and trusted lets us down to such an extent our basic trust is destroyed. Walker describes what this feels like for a child:

> Try to get inside a child's experience: the essence of trusting, and knowing that you matter, is the belief that when someone throws you up in the air they will catch you; that when you are frightened someone will comfort you; and those that matter most to you will not go away and leave you. What then, if instead you find yourself hitting the wall, or falling to the floor; or if the person who should provide comfort is the one who frightens you the most; or if you find yourself abandoned? When that happens, your small world becomes senseless; there is no one to tell: your potential protector has become your actual abuser. As a child you have no way of understanding any of this. You are left struggling to make sense of the senseless, when you are already hurt and utterly betrayed. Additionally your abuser probably blames you or threatens you. You are left feeling insignificant, bad, frightened and alone, with precious little self-esteem.

Life is dangerous. There is no comfort. Fears are intensified, and anxieties justified . . . everything and everyone becomes unpredictable. The world as the child knows it becomes unsafe, while any world that is perceived beyond the immediate one is distant and unattainable.

(1992: 95)

The experience of betrayal can make it difficult to form meaningful relationships. It generates a fear of intimacy in adulthood. People become isolated, feeling utterly alone, unable to risk loving or even getting close to another person. At times, it feels all too much and suicidal thoughts swirl seductively through the mind.

The shattering of innocence and curiosity

One of the gifts children give is their innocence and child-like way of viewing the world. Amilie looked up through her fringe with big eyes and said with such seriousness, 'I am four and I am sad'. I replied, 'I am old, and I am sad sometimes too'. She smiled before returning to her play. Her father explained, 'Yesterday we stayed with some friends who have just had puppies. Amilie fell in love with one and informed us, "I am staying here now but you and Mamma can come and visit if you like". She was heartbroken when we left'. Her innocence and curiosity remained intact despite this loss and I hope her innocence and curiosity remain for a long time to come. It is these endearing child-like qualities that get smashed almost beyond repair through sexual abuse. Contemporary psychodynamic therapy fosters a curiosity that repairs (to some extent) damage done through sexual abuse. It also engenders a capacity to play and a recovery of a sense of self and agency often lost in the breaking of innocence by abuse.

Trauma's impact on the therapist

In working with trauma, especially sexual trauma, we need to listen, offering a safe space for a client's story to be heard and believed, and then listen again with an even greater intensity. Only if we can enter into these dark, cavernous depths will the client find an unconscious trust that has been so badly damaged and find ways of connecting with their enclaved psyche. This is, however, incredibly demanding where therapists themselves are likely to become traumatised to some degree. As in all helping professions, there is a risk of vicarious traumatisation.

Jim's story

Jim was a tough police sergeant working in a tough inner-city neighbourhood. He had seen pretty much everything and believed he was hardened to any event, and anyone needing support or counselling because of stress was weak. Jim was embarrassed explaining this to his counsellor, as he was off work with stress and his manager had made it compulsory that he seek help. Jim was resistant to the 'boo-hoo-hoo let's talk about your feelings' approach he thought counselling would be.

His presenting problem was that his cat had been run over in an accident and he found he couldn't stop crying. As we unpacked his story, it was full of losses from an early age. Therapy helped him see that the past links with the present, that unexpressed feelings don't have a shelf-life and still need expressing, that it is not 'stupid' to feel upset, and that there was another side to him 'split off' to protect that was caring and vulnerable.

Jim had built strong psychological defences and found a job with a hierarchy and a 'tough' image that he felt suited his personality. Getting in touch with the many stresses, traumas, and losses of his job – he recalled a harrowing traffic accident where his role was to pick up many body parts – he had slowly consumed all his emotional coping resources and had nothing left. The death of his cat was the final event pushing him into breakdown.

Therapy helped him see that he was normal, had experienced vicarious traumatisation, and that he needed to find new ways of coping. Jim had twelve sessions of therapy, which he described as 'the toughest thing I've ever done', and returned to work somewhat chastened. He also discovered he liked elderly people and had started volunteering at a local centre. A larger than life character, they loved him and this rebalanced his emotional life, giving him a different and affirming engagement with people in need. Yet therapists don't always see this in their own emotional life, in the way they so clearly can in their clients.

Orange (2010) believes it is vital we allow ourselves to experience the trauma of our clients. She draws on the work of Jewish philosopher, Emmanuel Levinas. Writing out of his experiences in a prisoner-of-war camp, he believed that we need to enter into the sufferings of another rather than defend ourselves from them, as Orange would say through our theoretical stance or by diagnosing and categorising. We need to let the trauma speak, and in this we bear witness to trauma as an experience, living out in the life of the client. We, too, are never untouched, as we all have our own traumas to bear and we, too, have always wanted someone to believe in us, in our trauma.

Trauma is a living memory rather than an event and this needs to be replaced. Traumatised clients will elicit traumatised transference processes with the potential for forms of re-enactment (an unconscious repeating of previous unhelpful patterns), which are damaging to the client and the therapist. After one challenging client who took me beyond my abilities, into an abyss, I was caught up in just such a re-enactment. It took me several years to fully recover my confidence as a therapist and re-think my practice. In this context, supportive and challenging clinical supervision is vital. At that stage, I wish I had read the work of Bromberg (2001, 2006), who offers innovative and valuable theoretical insights and clinical practices when working with these extremely challenging transference and counter-transference dynamics. Dissociation is a normal interpersonal process that can be a source of creativity and a healthy way of protecting the person. It becomes pathological when it impinges on our reflective capacity and splits the mind from the self. Bromberg (1996) highlights the need for the therapist to work with their own dissociations and see how these are potentially re-enacted in psychodynamic therapy. Such an enabling therapeutic process can lead to the client's recovery even if this is a slow, painstaking process.

Summary

Working with trauma and abuse accounts for a large part of the work we do as therapists. It is easy to underestimate the pervasive impact of such events in a client's life. Contemporary psychodynamic therapists work with such skills as transference, counter-transference, projective identifications, co-created intersubjectivity, enactments, ruptures, and dissociations (see Chapters 13 and 14), all of which is demanding work requiring a greater knowledge as well as supportive and insightful supervision.

Reflective questions

Have you identified and dealt with trauma in your own life?

If applicable, how did you find therapy helpful and how did it enable you to address such issues?

What are your fears about working with clients who have been sexually abused?

Looking at research

The following research papers outline the difficulty of using RCTs in cases of sexual abuse and complex trauma. These cases often get excluded on the basis that there are pre-existing issues, such as abuse, that could affect the research focus.

Price, J., Hilsenroth, M., Callahan, K., Petretic-Jackson, P. and Bonge, D. (2004) A pilot study of psychodynamic psychotherapy for adult survivors of childhood sexual abuse, *Clinical Psychology & Psychotherapy*, 11(6): 369–438.

Schottenbauer, M., Glass, C., Arnkoff, D. and Gray, S. (2008) Contributions of psychodynamic approaches to treatment of PTSD and trauma: a review of the empirical treatment and psychopathology literature, *Psychiatry*, 71(1): 13–34.

Spermon, D., Darlington, Y. and Gibney, P. (2010) Psychodynamic psychotherapy for complex trauma: targets, focus, applications, and outcomes, *Psychology Research and Behavior Management*, 3: 119–127.

13

Foundational skills for practice

In this and the next chapter, we will examine what happens in therapy. We will begin with assessment and formulation, before moving through developing a therapeutic alliance, building empathy, understanding complex past relationships, using transference, counter-transference, projective-identification, engaging with intersubjectivity, working with resistance, dreaming dreams, bearing witness and suffering, working with spirit/soul, the importance of faith, and ending the relationship. I have highlighted key skills throughout (McWilliams 2004; Lemma 2016; Howard 2017).

If I were a newly minted therapist, or therapist in training (psychodynamic, integrative, or otherwise), having read the last twelve chapters, I would be terrified even imagining sitting in a counselling room with a real client. Now knowing all the things that could possibly be going wrong, or what could be happening at conscious and unconscious levels, would leave me feeling bewildered, if not a little scared. The good news is that this feeling soon passes, if we take some simple steps. It is good to be a little afraid, just not terrified or paralysed. As Bion famously said,

> In every consulting room there ought to be two rather frightened people: the patient and the psycho-analyst. If they are not, one wonders why they are bothering to find out what everyone knows.

> (1990: 5)

The whole purpose of dynamic therapies is to work with the unconscious, which means we never know what will emerge. Bion's playful comment gives due regard for the importance of the role we undertake and the tasks that lie ahead. Now that we have got over the fright of having a client in the room, what do we do with them? This is the moment when we turn theory into practice.

Here is a real-life first session with 'Terry'. Like real life, it is not a perfect example, but it shows what goes on and from this we can draw out what psychodynamic techniques are at work, before exploring other techniques from later sessions. Throughout this chapter, I will draw on the case of Terry to help illuminate each skill.

Terry's story – the first session

Terry rang asking for counselling, having been recommended by his business mentor's therapist. We agreed a date and time, and I gave directions to my home (where I have a room dedicated to my counselling practice). I stated I do not have a waiting room so it was important he came at the agreed time. I explained I do an initial assessment session to see if I am the right type of therapist for his needs and the fee for this was £50.

Terry arrived five minutes late, saying he had found it difficult to get out of the office, not wanting to tell anyone where he was going and why he was leaving early (even though he was the CEO). He sat down on the small settee opposite me and blurted out, 'My mentor sent me'. I replied, I wondered what it was that his mentor saw that made him 'send' Terry for therapy. Terry said that he greatly respected the wisdom of this older man and, over several years, his advice had always been helpful. I noted he had not answered my question. I remained silent, respectfully waiting for Terry to tell me more but in his own time. There was an embarrassing silence until Terry said accusingly, 'Aren't you going to ask me some questions?' I replied, 'I am still waiting and wanting to hear why you are here, although I understand it is often difficult to know where to begin'.

I noted that Terry's body language changed, he relaxed a little into the settee. He looked up and smiled, 'On the way here I was practising what I was going to say but now I'm here . . . (pause) . . . my wife and I are having some difficulties. My mentor says it's probably my temper'. He looked up as if seeking reassurance, seeming much younger, more like a boy than the man seated in front of me. 'I've never hit her but I get so angry, I say awful things'. I replied, 'I wonder if there are some awful things that you need to share with me in this confidential space'. He continued, 'I don't know where this rage comes from. But I can see how it is affecting Julie'. 'Tell me about Julie',' I asked.

There followed a long story about how he had met Julie (in her late twenties), through a mutual friend following an acrimonious divorce. Terry (in his late thirties) was single and had put all his energies into building up his management consultancy firm. At this point, Terry asked about a cost–benefit analysis for the therapy including the number of sessions, what it would cost, and how it would resolve his problems. My reply was that Terry was dealing with his anxiety about seeing me by trying to manage a transaction rather than a relationship. Terry laughed, 'I do that all the time!'

'Tell me more about your family of origin', I asked. At this point, Terry became visibly upset, saying his mother had died two years ago. He missed her and hadn't realised how much it would 'change things'. 'Change things?', I echoed. 'Well, it was Mum who kept everyone together and Dad isn't really managing on his own. My brother wants a family conference. He lives the closest, but his wife doesn't like my dad and makes that very clear. Not that I blame her, he's not a very nice man. My sister is weird'. Terry laughed in a derisive way saying, 'She's into crystals and healing energies and lives in Glastonbury. You don't believe any of that nonsense, do you?', he asked. I replied, 'I believe your mum's death has shaken something deep within you that you can't figure out in your head. But it's left you angry and feeling out of control, which links to events in the past'. Terry looked as if a light had been switched on but we were close to finishing our 50-minute assessment session. Terry said this session had been revealing and so wanted to come for a further six sessions. I explained that we could work for six sessions and then review with the possibility of open-ended therapy as required.

During the session, I was thinking about the 'fit' between us, as well as being alert to my 'free-floating attention' trying to catch the occasional glimpses of the unconscious at work. My working hypothesis was Terry's anger was, in part, unexpressed grief at the loss of his mother. The other part came from his past, and relationships within it, especially with his distant but demanding father. This latter part was informed more by what he did not say and the tone of voice when he did. Terry's defences were to exist in a psychological split, either by dismissing or denigrating others (sister) or idealising them (mentor). There was also an element of calculation (cost–benefit analysis) and, as we shall see later, issues around money. My dynamic formulation (we shall explore this later) was that Terry had been 'let down' by important others and his unconscious feelings were surfacing, triggered by his mother's death. This led to the 'trial interpretation' I made at the end of the session.

Terry retrieved his cheque book from his case and said, '£50 a session, that's a bit steep'. I replied saying some therapists charged less and others more, and then asked him what his salary was. He replied, 'Roughly £100,000'. My response was that he could easily afford my fees so maybe he was telling me what he couldn't afford was the emotional cost of the therapy. Terry smiled sheepishly as if he had been caught out like a naughty schoolboy and handed me a cheque for £350 to pay for our agreed sessions.

The question I needed to ask was, 'Is Terry suitable for a psychodynamic approach?' You've read the exchanges, so what do you think? Some potential clients are not. If Terry had stayed resolutely in the present, distant from his emotions, existing solely in his cognitions and calculations, I would not have worked with him and would instead have referred him to a colleague who worked integratively. Integrative therapists often draw on cognitive-based and person-centred approaches, which could help Terry even if he were not suitable for a psychodynamic way of working.

When clients are not ready for therapy – four key reasons

With Terry, as with all clients, we need to ask whether therapy is right for them. There are other reasons why we might not work with clients at all, or the work comes to a rapid conclusion.

First, *for some people seeking therapy, we are the wrong person.* Being blunt – our age, race, gender, class, religion, sexual orientation, or theoretical stance are not what they expected, or wanted. Clients seeking therapy for the first time find themselves overwhelmed by choices. An internet search for a specific town will return a frankly alarming variety of therapists claiming to work with almost any client group and using a bewildering range of techniques. Someone expecting a warm, immediately empathic, here-and-now focused therapist might struggle with a more restrained, waiting without words (including space for silences) therapist, and vice versa.

Traditionally, psychodynamic therapists are as neutral as possible, revealing little, whilst still being present for the client. With the internet, this is no longer possible. My university role is public and a great deal of information is available online. This includes the fact that I write about the interface between religion, spirituality, psychoanalysis, and psychotherapy (Ross 2010, 2016c, 2016d). One client I saw through a referral from a university colleague said at the end of 16 sessions, 'I thought you would be more religious', despite the fact this had not been the focus of our work. Knowing something of my background did not stop us from working effectively together, but it might for some. It is important that through assessment (we will come to this later in this chapter), we can identify the right fit between client and therapist.

Clare's story

Clare came into the session looking a little sheepish and started the session saying, 'I told my best friend I was seeing a therapist and she Googled you. I hadn't done that before as I took you on trust from Sarah who recommended you. I didn't realise you were . . .' listing a number of things I have done and work I have published. I wondered with Clare whether this had changed her perception of me. She felt she had found the 'right' therapist but was a little surprised about what she had subsequently discovered, though this is more fuel to stoke the therapy fire. Clients' transference (see later section in this chapter) begins before and during their first contact with us. When they meet us, we become subject to all sorts of projections, which can give us insight into their inner world. Clare's projections were positive, which revealed her tendency to idealise male authority figures but at the cost of giving away her agency.

Second, *for some seeking therapy, it is not the right time*. Bereavement is such a simple word but it is a process that contains multiple layers of devastating loss, immense sadness, overwhelming pain, utter rawness and rage, even futility (Lewis 1961). It can be seen coming from a long way in the distance with the diagnosis of a terminal illness or arrive like an unexpected hurricane that obliterates all it meets; the effects are the same. So clients seeking therapy who have been recently bereaved may not be ready for an in-depth examination of their psyche. They would be better in the short term with supportive listening or counselling in a safe, contained space to pour out their grief.

Therapy is hard work, it stirs up painful material, it strips away our defences often revealing what we fear, it connects us with powerful emotions, it brings out our dependence and, when it's all over, a new kind of loss. Therapy is something we need to be ready for, even if it takes us in unexpected directions, and for some it is too soon, or sadly in a few cases too late.

Sam's story

Sam was referred to me because of my background as a minister of religion (Baptist). Sam worked for a Christian organisation but was off work with stress. They were willing to pay for her to see a professional who would take account of a faith background.

I saw her for three sessions and, in the third, she explained why she was not coming back. In the previous session, she had asked me to pray for her. I interpreted this as her asking for additional help, so I wondered what it was I was missing. Sam hinted she had a traumatised past, leaving me with the impression it was some form of sexual abuse. The Church had become a new family for her, where her faith was about the future, and 'All that stuff from the past had been dealt with'. My sense was that Sam's faith, while very real, was also a defence and it seemed she was not willing to explore how the past shapes the present and the future. I may have been able to help Sam, but she left.

The luxury of choosing a therapist only occurs in private practice. In an NHS context, you get who you get, although all therapists should be willing to work with issues of difference and diversity, both their own and those of others (Wheeler 2006). For Sam, it was just the wrong time. When we experience a profound loss, such as a death or divorce, the grief can be like having a wound opened up, leaving us bleeding and raw, waiting for the body to heal and the skin to knit together, leaving an indelible scar. This also happens to the psyche. Having the lid ripped off and exposing the contents inside is a frightening process that can take us to the edge of breakdown. We can peer in, but we quickly slam the lid back down for fear of disturbing what is within.

Third, *sometimes we think we want to change but discover through therapy that we don't*. Sean Scully is a contemporary Irish-British painter (now based in New York) whose large abstracts composed of lines and squares communicate at a primitive level, just like great poetry. I once stood transfixed, gazing longingly at his work displayed in a Grand Canal palazzo, Venice. There is an unspoken precision about them as he appears to re-work themes again and again. One of those themes is grief and loss. Following the tragic death of his young son, he went to see a therapist for a time, who eventually told him to go and paint instead. Scully discovered he liked himself just as he was and it was more cathartic to paint.

Fourth, *potential clients may not be suitable for a psychodynamic therapy because they know that they want an alternative form of therapy*, either a cognitive approach with specific targets and tasks, or a person-centred approach focusing on the here-and-now relationship. In this regard, integrative therapists or counselling psychologists offer a better fit, having a wide range of theoretical ideas and skills they can utilise, which is the great strength of these approaches (Finlay 2016). Other potential clients may be put off by the time-limited nature of therapies offered through the NHS, university, college, and voluntary counselling services. Whilst much creative therapeutic work can be done in six sessions, it can limit how we work with deeper, long-standing issues.

Kerry's story

Kerry was referred to me by her GP. She instinctively knew that she needed more than the six sessions (available through the university counselling service) and that her parents were willing to pay the fees.

We worked together for two years enabling her to get a greater awareness of who she was and why she got caught up in complex relationships with girlfriends and boyfriends, romantic or otherwise. When these relationships inevitably broke down, Kerry became depressed, withdrew, and stopped doing any academic work. She came to understand that her depleted sense of self meant she projected her hopes (and fears) into each new relationship, not feeling that she had anything to offer. It was as if she had no 'psychic skin' to protect herself. This linked with patterns in her family and her parents' divorce. When her father left, she no longer felt special to anyone, as her mother always favoured her younger sister.

We stopped working together in her final year following a period when she survived a relationship break-up but, rather than getting depressed, continued working – she had made satisfactory progress, she had developed a 'psychic skin'. Kerry knew she still had therapeutic work to do but felt she had come a long way and wanted to try being independent. She sent me a card of the day of her graduation, celebrating her success and hopeful about her future.

All clients benefit from being listened to at a level and depth greater than anything they have ever experienced. Such therapist–client relating forms the core of the therapeutic relationship, which recent studies suggest is paramount to offering the client a way of regaining, in Kerry's case, an enduring 'psychic skin'. Psychodynamic therapists construct the therapist–client relationship in a very particular way, beginning with thinking about the client even before assessment; such a skill is fundamental to this form of therapy.

The structure of psychodynamic therapy

The structure of open-ended psychodynamic therapy consists of three or four stages. A four-stage model includes: assessment leading to formulation (1–2 sessions); a beginning phase that involves building a therapeutic alliance (1–6 sessions); a middle phase that involves working with unconscious processes, while working through core issues using transference and counter-transference, working with resistance (1–∞); and an ending phase (ideally negotiated based on the length of time working together) sometimes called 'termination', which to my mind has rather unfortunate connotations. Time-limited approaches vary greatly in the number of sessions, which we shall explore in Chapter 14.

Even before the client walks through the door for the first assessment session, dynamic therapists need to be able to do something that is crucially important and deeply impactful. This is to be able to carve out a safe space or place for the client to enter into. Clients' recollections of good therapy are often about something that was attended to at an unconscious level. They felt wanted in and welcomed into this therapeutic space, unconsciously

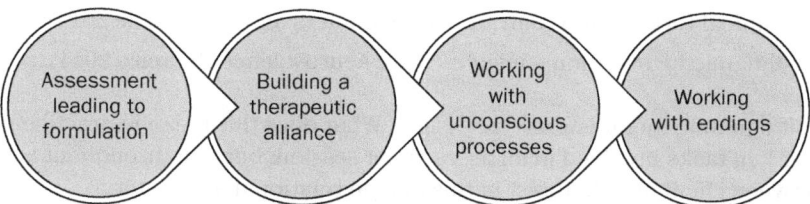

Figure 13.1 Structure of psychodynamic therapy

communicating that this had been lacking from their past (Grosz 2013). This fits with the wealth of research evidence drawn from infant development (Chapters 9 and 10). As the mother carries her baby in the womb, she is also carrying it in her mind. Her hopes, joys, anxieties, and fears mingle in a potent cocktail for a placenta-fed psyche of the yet-to-be-born person. The trauma of entry into this world is overcome by being touched, held, wanted, gazed at, and attuned, and exists in the memory of the infant. Often these experiences are absent and explain why the adult person is now entering therapy.

Therapy begins in the mind of the therapist, operating in the psyche, not only as a place of safety but as a place of welcome. In Winnicott's terms, it offers a holding environment or, in Bion's terms, a contained function (Abram 2013; Levine and Brown 2013). The therapeutic space offers a place where anything can be thought or said, free from criticism and judgement, though not without challenge. It offers confidentiality (with limits identified); a deep listening to the spoken and unspoken; and clarity about the way therapy operates, psychologically and practically. It allows both parties to gain trust and allows informed consent to occur, an issue that therapists have overlooked for far too long (Danchev and Ross 2013).

Let's look now at each of the four stages of psychodynamic therapy, as detailed in Figure 13.1.

Assessment

Like two sides of a coin, assessment and formulation form the basic currency of a psychodynamic approach. Whilst Anna Freud pioneered a form of diagnostic assessment (Midgley 2013), this evolved to become more dynamic in nature. Many terms are used to capture this initial meeting before the therapy begins in earnest. These include:

- assessment (Coltart 1992; Lemma 2016);
- evaluation (Cabaniss et al. 2011);
- assessment consultations (Hobson 2016);
- psychodynamic interviewing (Gabbard 2010);
- assessment and formulation (Howard 2017);
- dynamic formulation (Lemma 2016);
- psychodynamic formulation – looking beneath the surface (Leiper 2014);
- problem formulation and 'storying' (Finlay 2016);
- psychoanalytic case formulation (McWilliams 1999);

- case or clinical formulation (Safran 2012; Summers and Martindale 2013); and
- psychodynamic formulation – insights from neuroscience (Shapiro 2014).

So what is it dynamic therapists are assessing? What does this mean in practice? There are a number of key tasks involved in an assessment session, but key throughout is the unspoken 'fit' between client and therapist in this unique relational encounter.

Key assessment tasks and skills

1. Asking the right questions to get the right answers (illustrated by my work with Terry, who we met at the outset of this chapter, highlighted in italics)

What does the client want from therapy?
Terry wasn't sure. He was doing what another 'father figure' suggested. It was something to do with his temper. He recalled seeing a look in his son's eyes when he was shouting at his wife. This caused him to stop, but stirred feelings he couldn't quite identify.

Why now? What has precipitated the desire for therapy?
Terry realised his anger was getting out of control and was disturbed by feelings he knew were both familiar and remote. He wanted to stop something getting worse.

What is the client's present problem/issue and am I equipped, through training or experience, to deal with this?
My reflection as a therapist was centred on the fact that I have worked with male clients and anger issues before. I was alert to any disclosures of physical violence towards his wife or children and the possibility of the need to refer the matter to the appropriate authorities. This was an issue I talked about in supervision.

When the client tells me their story, what doesn't fit or make sense?
I found myself reflecting on the questions, 'Who was he really angry with?', 'What area of his identity was feeling most under threat?'

What is the client not telling me, but hinting at?
The wider family connections seemed strained but felt more like emotional gaps in a story, the significance of which was unclear. He seemed like a lost child but as an adult could not admit this to himself.

Does the client listen to the questions I am asking, or do they tell me what they think I want to hear?
At first it felt like Terry was telling me what he thought I wanted to hear. Although, as I made connections with what he was saying and probed further, he began to say more about himself that felt less rehearsed and more honest.

When I draw attention to an aspect of the past within the present issue, can the client make a connection either rationally or emotionally?
I made a trial link between the past and the present. 'You are telling me you get very angry, explode verbally, but then feel remorse and powerlessness. Can you think of a time in your past when you had similar feelings about being powerless?' Terry connected to an event in his childhood when he was forced to leave a public school he loved and attended the local state school (as his father's business had got into financial difficulties).

Is the client able to talk about uncomfortable issues – for instance, suicidal feelings, self-harm, sexual experiences, or addictions? Given these issues are often experienced as shameful, the therapist needs to be sensitive in the way these are raised. They may need to gently tease out the information from the clues offered by the client.

Terry looked ashamed when he described his verbal aggression. I was alert to how I framed questions and the tone with which they were expressed to avoid shaming him further. Terry volunteered that even when he felt at his worst, he had never had suicidal thoughts or feelings.

Are there spiritual/religious resources or traditions the client might want to draw on?

Terry had a faith background, which was both a resource and an obstacle, as this compounded feelings of guilt after his verbal onslaughts, leaving him feeling a failure.

What do I 'see' in the client and 'sense' about their inner world? This can come in the form of an image or an association that has its origins in the unconscious becoming conscious. How do I envision who they could become?

If I am entirely honest, while with some clients I have a sense of 'seeing', Terry felt very closed in and I could not see much. There was a fleeting image of an oyster (that I hoped would contain a pearl) but in that moment all I saw was the grooved callous shell.

What thoughts, feelings, or emotions are stirred in me, experienced in my mind and body?

I formed the impression in my mind of a frightened, lonely boy grieving the loss of his mother and angry with his father (for reasons I did not yet know).

2. *Starting a collaborative process*. Lemma (2016) identifies the components of an analytic frame and attitude as consistency, reliability, neutrality, anonymity, and abstinence, which contain the clinical work and establish a context for insight and interpretation. Each component is valuable but one of the changes in contemporary psychodynamic therapy has been a moving beyond focusing on insight, where fragments of thought and feeling come together like a mystery solved by Sherlock Holmes in a verbal denouement. There is a move towards a co-constructed event of shared discovery and growth involving 'a fusion of horizons in which both client and therapist come to a shared perspective on reality by allowing themselves to be influenced by one another . . . the only way to truly understand our clients is to enter into their relational worlds and play out various scenarios with them in an unconscious way' (Safran 2012: 78f.). Developing a formulation is very helpful but not the sole *raison d'être* of assessment. We need to focus as much on the on-going dynamic in the therapy itself so that it becomes a continuous process, rather than a series of steps in which formulation shapes more accurate interpretations, which influence insight and offers the possibility of change through the relationship. In my clinical experience, we need both, and part of the skill a therapist develops is knowing, for each client, when to offer or encourage insight and how to develop the relationship in the room with the client, and in what balance. There are no easy answers to this.

3. *Searching for psychological mindedness* (again illustrated by my work with Terry, highlighted in italics). Coltart (1992) believes assessment is the place to discover if the client is psychologically minded. Can they make sense of a link between their past and their present? Do they reveal a curiosity to know more about themselves?

It took a little time in the first session with Terry to tease this out. I was not sure at first, especially when he asked for a cost–benefit analysis for the therapy; however, once we moved to his family context, he began to make links about the roots of his anger, which offered me some hope he could develop greater awareness into himself. Ironically, having thought he would only need six sessions, we worked together for two years and this only finished because I moved away from London to take up an academic post.

I am constantly amazed at the number of people that insist the past is the past and has no bearing on the present. The partner of a client who had been sexually abused, when she told him what we were working on said, 'You're not still going on about that? That was years ago. And anyway he's dead, so what's the point?' This betrays a lack of psychological mind-edness and, sadly, an absence of empathy. Determining if someone is psychologically minded is a skill that takes time to hone, so inevitably we will make mistakes and discover clients that initially seemed promising but fail to move beyond a superficial level. Let me introduce a note of caution. Being psychologically minded is not the same as 'thinking like me', which can make us feel initially comfortable with a client but admit the risk that they have similar blind-spots to us, offering scope for unconscious collusion.

4. Building a therapeutic frame

Angie's story

Angie moved to a new house. The whole of her life was still packed in boxes when her grandsons arrived for the weekend. They were not concerned there was little furniture in the house, or what they were going to sleep on, their single-minded focus was on finding their box of Lego. They wanted to build their own home.

How we build a therapeutic frame varies from setting to setting, and therapist to therapist (Gray 1994; Lemma 2016). In psychodynamic working, it is vital to set boundaries, as so often it is at the edges of the frame we discover the inner world of our clients. Building the frame includes paying attention to:

- location (a room that is comfortable and private, including access to a toilet);
- timing (hour, day, frequency);
- arriving exactly on time (many private practices do not have a waiting area);
- cancelling sessions (notice period, charges);
- notice of therapist's breaks;
- fees, payment, and financial transactions;
- managing expected or unexpected breaks (pregnancy, illness);
- contact outside the therapy room (shopping, conferences); and
- future contact or returning to therapy.

Having worked with a therapist for four years, eight years later I sought to resume therapy for a short period due to an unexpected event. My former therapist declined because, in moving towards retirement, she was neither taking on new clients nor seeing previous clients. I felt disappointed but valued the clarity of her thinking. In hindsight, in my mind I thought this would be 'short', but my unconscious may have had other plans. My previous therapist, in 'holding' this aspect of the frame, enabled me to find a new therapist more appropriate for where I was now.

5. *Listening for a 'cautionary tale'.* A cautionary tale is found in folk stories or fairy tales and used to warn, or 'caution', the reader about something that could happen but has not happened yet if they break some rule (or enter some forbidden forest). I used to make up bedtime stories for my daughter, Hannah, about a naughty schoolgirl called 'Horrible Hannah'. In these stories, she would get up to all kinds of mischief in various adventures but there was always a lesson to be learnt at the end.

Likewise, Lemma and colleagues introduced the idea of the 'cautionary tale' in Dynamic Interpersonal Therapy (DIT) (Lemma et al. 2011), which applies to all therapies. Clients tell us their cautionary tale and we need to hear them. When the client says, 'It ended badly with the last therapist', what I should hear is, 'And it might end badly here too', rather than any appeal to a saviour-complex or narcissism, 'But I am not that therapist, I will do things better'. Having now discovered cautionary tales, I realise these are more common than I had previously recognised.

6. *Doing a risk assessment.* In many agencies or placement contexts, this is an essential requirement; however, therapists in private practice often pay less attention to this than is wise. My practice is to do this at the end of an assessment so that I have a fuller picture, one that, for instance, sets any suicidal thoughts and feelings in context. These need to be talked about openly to discover the extent of the client's suicidal thinking, whether they have made any plans and whether they would tell you if they were going to act. Severe forms of depression can unexpectedly plunge a client into such a dark place – in that moment, their logic convinces them that everyone would be better off if they were dead. For others, it is a desperate cry for help, which sometimes goes unheard.

A sad story

While I was attached to the chaplain's department of a psychiatric hospital, I saw a person to help them work out what help they needed. After an acrimonious divorce, she discovered her ex-husband's younger partner was now pregnant. She felt very angry, utterly betrayed, and hoped her ex would 'pay for his crimes'. I asked if she was feeling depressed or suicidal, but she said 'no'. I suggested she visit her GP, who had given her anti-depressants but whom she had not seen for six months, to ask for a referral for counselling. We agreed I would see her in a month's time.

Three weeks later, I received a call asking me to attend her funeral, as she had committed suicide. She had not gone to her GP, despite my and her family's encouragement. On the surface, she appeared to be doing well, seeming far less depressed than she had been.

Risk assessment is important but it cannot prevent a person determined to take their own life (Reeves 2010).

7. *Obtaining informed consent*. This topic is missing from most psychodynamic texts (Howard 2017 is an exception). What is it and why is it necessary? Consider an analogy. Preparing for a routine operation, I had a pre-meeting with the nurse who explained the procedures and risks I needed to know before going ahead. She said there was a 1 in 10 chance it was cancer and a 1 in 20,000 chance I could die. Such statistics are sobering but, duly informed, one can give consent. What are the conditions for informed consent in contemporary psychodynamic therapy?

An academic colleague who described himself as 'a regular consumer of therapy', told me that he was not convinced any therapist should simply be taken on trust, shrouded in therapeutic mystique and hiding behind arcane language. He made the point that therapy can do people harm as well as good. He believes clients should know this in advance and an assessment session provides the opportunity to explain how dynamic therapies work with unconscious processes that by their nature are not known but can be seen in the use of transference.

Therapy can generate uncomfortable memories, thoughts, and feelings – so it is not for the faint-hearted. Relationships are relationships, they are not easy, and like most things in life, they need to be worked at. Clients also need to know the nature and scope of confidentiality (see later in this chapter), including the fact that the process of therapy will be talked about in clinical supervision with another person (or group). They need to know that every reputable therapist is accountable to their professional body and works within an ethical framework (BACP), a code of ethics and conduct (British Psychological Society) or ethical principles, and a code of professional conduct (UKCP). Additionally, as I am an academic and a writer, I ask if I can have their consent to draw on material that arises in sessions in a suitably anonymised way, as seen in the vignettes of this book.

Formulation

What information does the client need to make a formulation as a rough working hypothesis to guide the therapist through the twists and turns of another's psyche? At best, a formulation explains:

- why the client's psychological balance has become upset;
- how problems have developed (in their inner and outer worlds);
- a focus for the course of therapy;
- the potential consequences of change (positive and negative); and
- the possibility of realising that change.

Formulation is like an ordinance survey map for therapy, which gets re-negotiated once we are in the actual terrain. Like all hill-walking, the unpredictable factor is the weather, which influences the choices we make. (A January walk planned for the exciting but hair-raising Crib Gough route to the summit of Snowdon was abandoned due to sub-zero temperatures and wind-driven snow. We still made the summit via the Pyg track but it was not what we had planned.) Formulations are great plans that need translating in the unpredictable climate of another's psyche. While engaged in an assessment, we mentally create a reflective space so we can build a formulation using six simple steps. These are easier to describe than do, so it is a skill that evolves with clinical experience. (A more detailed step-by-step process can be found in Lemma [2016].)

1. *Identifying the problem*. This is not always the presenting issue, which is often the tip of the iceberg, above the surface. Psychodynamic therapy works best when it addresses what lies below the waterline. What is their core issue that causes them pain? This will take several attempts, each getting closer to the core like peeling an onion where tears – real or metaphorical – are often involved.

2. *Exploring how this impacts the person's sense of self*. People don't always know the self they present to others. Therapy offers the opportunity to act as a mirror where the person can see who they are, even if they don't like what they see.

3. *Identifying the context of the problem*. Everybody's context is different. Helpful information includes, to name a few: the make-up of the family of origin; the person's place or role within it; relationships with siblings; early traumas; significant losses; experience at school; and physical and mental health. Each therapist makes their own list as to what they believe to be the best questions to ask, although this can vary from client to client.

4. *Examining the most significant relationships (past and present) and how the client sees their self in relation to these*. At this point, you are trying to get a glimpse of the client's internal world and what insight the client has about this. For most clients this is a parent, or grandparent, though in my work with twins it is often the other twin, especially with lone twins (Woodward 1998).

5. *Identifying what gets in the way of relationships*. What defences does the client use to avoid psychic pain? In my work as an honorary therapist at the university counselling service, I worked primarily with doctoral students. In every case they used intellectual, rational, problem-solving defences to try and understand their emotional pain and confusion. What shocked them was understanding that a skill in which they were accomplished did not always diminish feeling emotional pain, or allow another part of themselves to receive much-needed help.

6. *Focusing areas to work on*. What do you and they hope might be achieved and can this be put into words?

Julia's story

One client, Julia, came because of difficulties in her relationships. She found that she wanted more and more from them until people rejected her as too demanding. Julia also said she wanted to address her weight issues and hoped therapy would help her lose weight. Bearing in mind this 'cautionary tale' (see earlier in the chapter) and the possibility that Julia would expect more and more of me and that I might let her down, I said that I could not work this issue and there might be better cognitive-based therapies that could make this the focus of the work. If I had agreed, I believed I would have been setting myself up for failure. Julia, however, insisted on turning to me for therapy. We therefore worked on this dynamic as she continued.

Julia discovered as a child she felt she had never been given enough and was 'replaced' when her sister was born. This came out early in the therapy when I asked about the age difference between her and her sister. Julie replied, 'One year, eleven months, and six days'.

By taking these different strands of information, we can build a formulation that covers the key psychodynamic needs of the client and how the therapy might progress. A formulation is only a working hypothesis, one that needs continual revision. Too definitive, it can become a straitjacket that robs the therapy of its dynamic creativity (Bollas 1992; Coltart 1992; Parsons 2000). Too diffuse, the therapy can drift into a collusive maze and conceptual confusion. This drift is unhelpful, so therapists find their own way of working in this crucial assessment formulation phase. Some are clearly structured, believing that clients need to know a sufficient amount in order to make an informed choice (Gabbard 2010). Others are much more unstructured, waiting to see what the client brings (Hobson 2016). Still others adopt an intersubjective stance that sees the assessment as a co-constructed event where the client waits for a moment something happens, an intuitive flash of insight, that enables the therapist to feel they can work well with this client. As a general principle, I would adopt an approach that is as loosely structured as possible while covering key areas and directly answering the client's questions, while exploring what lies behind the question. I also explain that I ask more questions and give more information at assessment but, once therapy starts, I normally wait for the client to initiate our work.

Establishing a therapeutic alliance

With May (Chapter 3), Terry, and the many client stories told throughout this book, it is clear that in our work we seek to establish helpful ways of working together. The phrase commonly used to describe this, the 'therapeutic alliance', doesn't sound that exciting; yet, it is at the heart of all therapeutic work and one of the most researched aspects of therapy. Relating to people and forming an alliance with them is one of our most basic human actions, described by Fairbairn as 'relationship-seeking' (Scharff and Scharff 2005).

Bollas (1999) offers a poetic account when he traces the origins of the therapeutic alliance to life in the womb, mediated through the mother, influenced by the father, and expressed in Oedipal dynamics. Every new alliance has its origins in our earliest alliances (Chapters 9 and 10) and is hugely significant in establishing the foundations of who we are today. Each new therapeutic encounter offers the potential for repair, re-discovery, and renewal. This requires the therapist to be ever alert to what is emerging from the past, coming alive and being replayed in the live encounters contained in the counselling space.

Establishing a therapeutic alliance is deeply curative in itself, giving therapists the chance to do more than repair. A repair is about making good and restoring to the original condition. A wonderful aspect of dynamic therapies is that they also aim to facilitate psychic growth, to realise potential, to find new freedom and enter into new relationships. In Winnicottian terms (Kahr 2016), it offers a moving beyond a *false* self to an appreciation of the *true* self, in as far as we glimpse this from time to time.

Clients need to feel they can trust this new relationship with their therapist and form an alliance that allows further risk and trust to develop. One way of constructing an alliance is to identify a focus for the work helped by a clear formulation, offering a guide across the terrain of another's psyche. This is especially important in time-limited work (Coren 2010). Practice varies – some contemporary psychodynamic therapists explicitly identify this focus in conjunction with the client, while others have an implicit understanding that it will become clear in and through the on-going work. Whatever our formulation, this needs to be continually adapted and refined as more information emerges in the therapy as a way of attending to the alliance. As the client learns to trust, they can bring their resistance, memories, or connections that emerge 'as if' for the first time, sometimes coming through dreams and other associations.

Gracie's story

Gracie, one of my former students, now an experienced therapist whose clinical work I supervise, recalled her training and my supervision of trainees. The part that caused her most 'trauma' (I hope she was joking) was when she started with a new client. Here, I expected the students in the supervision group to offer a two- or three-sentence formulation 'off the cuff', without thinking about it too much. All my supervisees found this challenging, as do I, but all felt that it enabled them to really get into the client's world at a deeper level and form a strong alliance that could sustain the vital work.

After qualifying and practising as a therapist for several years, Gracie knocked on my door wanting to be supervised. 'I never thought I would utter these words', she said, 'but I miss doing those impromptu formulations'.

Fostering einfühlung

There are times in our life when we experience someone who makes us feel that everything will be okay. It is as if they see right through our defences, denials, hurts, and shame, touching us in a way that communicates we are not alone. This is what empathy feels like and traditionally it forms a core part of person-centred and integrative therapies (Finlay 2016), rather than psychodynamic therapy. This needs to be rectified. The German word used by Freud is 'einfühlung' (literally meaning empathy), which was often translated as sympathy or intuition by James Strachey, Freud's English translator. This blunts Freud's use of einfühlung to convey an intuitive insight or a depth of understanding of others. Since Freud, it has been adopted to account for a depth of feeling and entering into the lives of others (Kohut 1977). It enhances and becomes expressed in and through projective identification (Ogden 1986); it adds a new layer of authenticity into the dynamic relationship (Orange 2002).

Often clients report experiences of parents habitually being angry, sometimes frightening, and lacking in warmth and affection, which gives us insight into what they want – they long for warmth and affection but are concerned about being frightened or angry, within themselves and with others. Therapy enables these thoughts and feelings to be expressed through a relationship, which repairs damage already done with the hope it is before it becomes worse or, as study suggests, before it is passed on from one generation to another.

If I reflect on my four experiences of therapy, ranging from nine months (shortest on a weekly basis) to four years (longest, twice a week), and the four clinical supervisors (over the last 20 years), all of which offered me something valuable, there are two therapists and two supervisors that stand out. What makes them memorable is the quality of their empathy when I needed it. Similarly, clients search for a sense that this stranger, the therapist, can understand them and feel for them, until they can discover their own feelings for themselves. Just as a mother engages with a baby through gaze, voice, tone, smell, skin, touch, and milk/breast (see Chapter 9), this engagement communicates a profound sense of safety and primal nurture that we seek out in every caring or nurturing relationship. This is why some clients do not thrive in traditional expressions of psychoanalytic psychotherapy, with a largely silent therapist, making minimal interventions, increasing anxiety, and focused solely on the inner world. This is the advance of contemporary, non-traditional psychodynamic therapy.

Juggling triangles

(illustrated by my work with Terry, highlighted in italics)

Learning how to negotiate relationships is a lifetime's task. These often form triangular patterns based on what we are looking for in a relationship, the response we get from the other person, and how we then react. Clients often come to therapy because of relationship issues, with some awareness that it is their own reaction that is causing difficulty. Psychodynamic therapists see these encounters as offering clues to early relationships, the internal expectations generated by these relationships (existing in the psyche as internal objects) and the patterns established.

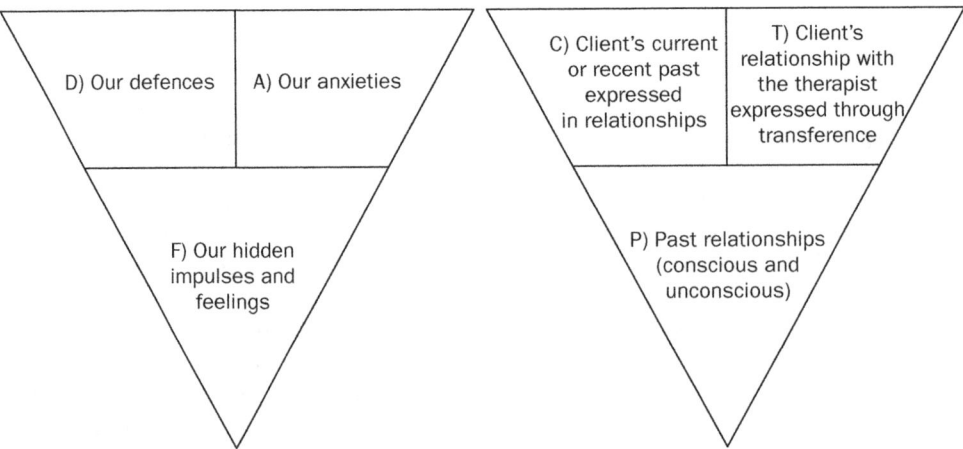

Figure 13.2 Malan's triangular models of conflict and persons

Malan (1979; Malan and Della Selva 2006) developed two triangular models to explain complex dynamic processes and the insights these offer to client work (see Figure 13.2). In the first model, Malan offered an inverted triangle where (D) locates our defences, (A) our anxieties and, because both our anxieties and defences have their origin in our hidden (often unconscious) impulses and feelings (F) such as anger, love, hate, and fear, these are located in the centre point at the bottom of the triangle. A client comes with a presenting problem, such as issues with a new manager at work, and this results in the client becoming defensive, overly alert to criticism, anxious about their performance, and depressed about their future in the company. Psychodynamic therapy using Malan's triangle of conflict helps us locate the origins of the hidden feelings, often in the past. Malan then introduced a triangle of persons to take this further. Psychodynamic therapy navigates each of these triangular relationships in a way that brings insight to the client, knowledge about the cause of symptoms, and new ways of thinking about past relationships and negotiating new relationships.

Thinking about Terry, his experiences of present relationships were three-fold: anger at his wife, irritation with his siblings, and pain caused by the loss of his mother. In the room, with me as his therapist, there was a deep ambivalence, spanning suppressed forms of anger (being five minutes late, 'Aren't you going to say something?') to grudging respect ('my mentor says you are very good and could help me get to the bottom of things').

Past relationships included the loss of his mother, and deep but unexpressed negative feelings about his father. I can't recall exactly what I said but my interpretation was along the lines, 'You are angry at your wife, you are angry with me (in a polite way), but I wonder if you are really angry about the fact it was your mum that died, and not your father. Now you are left with grief about this loss and many other losses in your past you have not yet fully recognised'. Terry acknowledged this as he recognised this unlocked something deeply buried in his childhood, which became the focus of the work.

The on-going negotiations around triangular relationships raise issues of inclusion and exclusion, power and authority, and dependence and autonomy that are always features of psychodynamic work. So in clinical work it is always helpful to have a 'triangle-in-mind'. When a client is telling us a story, we are connecting in our thinking others not yet present in the story in a flowing interchange of relationships. Then, as something or someone falls into place, the psychological narrative comes alive or enters a greater depth.

Transference and counter-transference

What do these forbidding-sounding terms mean? In brief compass, *transference* is when a client sees a therapist 'as if' they were an important figure from their past that they have feelings about (positive and negative). *Counter-transference* is the thoughts and feelings created in the therapist when encountering the conscious and unconscious of their client.

While these dynamic processes are more complicated than such brief summaries allow (Stefana 2017), the skill of a contemporary psychodynamic therapist is to identify and engage with them as a foundation for further intersubjective engagement. To do so requires drawing on our personal therapy where we have experienced these. While our client work is not a repeat of our own therapy (if it is, something has gone badly wrong), it means we know the psychic terrain. We exist in a landscape of latent emotion that takes us to the edge, and at times over the edge, into the abyss. Yet we come out alive, and more whole.

When I scramble up new peaks, such as the Cullins on the Isle of Skye, I hire a guide because I know they have done it before. They know the best routes and are alert to the ever-changing weather conditions as they are familiar with the local terrain. Similarly, being in therapy enables us to love, hate, bear ambivalence, project our fears but to receive them back in a containable way. We learn to love, trust, face our deepest fears, and be confronted with aspects of ourselves we do not like and have tried to hide. We thereby enter into the transferential processes of others with a map etched into our psyche. Before we went into therapy, we had a rich emotional life with its own issues. Yet there are wounds, blind spots, unhelpful patterns, and unconscious processes that need to be felt and thought about in therapy. After therapy, we continue learning and growing, set on a psychological trajectory but fuelled by our own desire to be fully the person we are. This means when clients encounter us, they are meeting someone whose psyche is alive and well, glistening with health, willing to engage creatively and bravely with whatever appears.

Focusing mainly on transference

As this is such a crucial area of psychodynamic practice, there are many books written on every aspect of transference and counter-transference. It is difficult to talk about one without the other, although historically Freud focused on transference. (Accessible overviews are to be found in Murdin [2009], Lemma [2016], and Howard [2017], while Person and Target offer valuable reflections on transference in their edited book based on Freud's *On Transference-Love* [2013].) Due to Oedipal and triangular dynamics (Chapters 8 and 11), we learn how to relate to others, sharing people and power, gaining acceptance and intimacy. So when a therapist connects a client with their past, it includes a whole cast of characters anxiously waiting to make an appearance. Through transference, a therapist can be experienced as a significant person from the client's past about whom they have powerful, unexpressed, or repressed feelings.

Tori's story

Tori became angry with me, which reflected her presenting issue about not getting the promotion at work she believed she deserved. 'I work harder and longer than anyone else. Then they just swan in and get the prize', she declared. I teased out what she meant by 'swan in' and 'prize'. Angrily she responded, 'you don't believe me either. That I can't do it. That I'm not clever enough'.

I was already thinking about which figure or figures from her past did not think she was good enough. Yet it seemed important to wait, to patiently endure her anger about what was the point of seeing me, as if I was not a good-enough therapist to 'sort out' her problems. These exchanges took place over three sessions of therapy. This space allowed her general, angry transference responses to male, authority figures to be more accurately located.

While Tori's transference was to a male authority figure, transference makes no distinction for age, gender, time, or any other form of difference. A female therapist can become seen 'as if' they were an abusive father or an idealised caring mother, to name a couple of possibilities.

Yet because of the dynamic nature of the relationship, the client moves in and out of multiple transferences. This is why keeping an eye on what has been called the 'total transference situation' (see next section) is vital. The work of the psychodynamic therapist is to tease out who or what this transferential figure might be. They could be seen 'as if' they were a tyrannical father, a safe mother, a longed-for lover, a difficult sibling, a harsh teacher, or some other figure variously idealised and denigrated, loved and hated.

One complication, however, is that clients can experience us through transference as a part-object. In object-relations thinking, the 'object' is a significant relationship that gets taken into the mind (and psyche) as something that is used to develop a sense of self. Thus, a 'part-object' is an aspect of one of these object-relations. In terms of transference, I could become a part-object abusive father and a part-object idealised mother. Here, the client experiences ambivalence at expressing anger as if I was that father and fears that, if they express this, they will lose the caring mother they need but are not able to fully access because their anger is getting in the way. Another complication is that it can be difficult to exactly match the transference phenomena being experienced in the counselling room with a whole person or a part-object, past or present. Yet we know something is going on because what we are experiencing with the client does not seem to fit. The words used don't match the feelings or actions that are expressed. They seem to be connecting things in a false, mistaken, or confused way. We, as therapists, often experience what you could call a 'transference muddle' when our normally clear thinking gets confused, or our feelings seem off-key.

Nina's story

As Nina told me her history of a warm, happy childhood, I experienced a glacial coldness that made me shiver. Yet there was neither an event nor any person to which this could be linked. Something was going on, but was it in my unconscious or her unconscious, or both intersubjectively, being experienced as a form of embodied counter-transference or projective identification? I couldn't work out what was happening, so I just sat with these uncomfortable feelings that didn't make sense. I would like to tell you that *this* event happened or Nina revealed *something* and it all made sense in terms of transference, that I could draw attention to something concrete through a neat interpretation. That did not happen. It just felt cold, and my mind was numb. Supervision, normally a reliable source of help, failed to offer any insight.

What I did do was offer to Nina a reflection about the process, with words like 'Sometimes things don't make sense, where our thoughts, feelings, or what we want to say are locked-up or frozen in the deep freeze of the psyche'. This shifted something in Nina but we never worked out exactly what it was.

The transferential process can be very confusing for clients experiencing it and the accompanying emotional intensity for the first, second, or even third time. It is also confusing for the therapist as they are feeling their way forward as if in the dark responding to glimmers of light. It has the potential to create misunderstandings, which need to be identified and worked through.

This is critical because, after the unconscious, the aspect of psychodynamic therapy that is most distinctive is working with transference and associated processes. It is so significant that Freud defined psychoanalysis as any form of investigation that recognised the importance of transference (and resistance) such that it becomes the basis of clinical work (1914b). Freud first developed transference as a therapeutic technique and viewed counter-transference as an interference to be dealt with in analysis (1910). He warned Jung and Ferenczi about it, but to no avail. Ferenczi, Klein, and many later analysts expanded the scope of thinking about transference to be more inclusive so Wallerstein (1990), writing about the common ground of psychoanalysis, re-stated the importance of transference and counter-transference (Stefana 2017) as part of the shared heritage of all psychoanalytic and psychodynamic perspectives.

At first glance, the technicalities of transference appear to be like a game of chess. It involves two people involved in a mental and emotional struggle involving: move and counter-move; attack and defence; sacrificing some aspects (pawns) to regain control; planning or intuition; noticing patterns that become repeated; and calculating multiple options. There is even a Freudian interpretation of chess where the drive is the desire of each player to take control of the Queen (mother) in order to attack or supplant the King (father) in a dramatic repeat of the Oedipal struggle. In reality, transference is very different and it is better experienced than theorised. When Freud began treating his own patients, his ever-curious scientific mind searched for a hypothesis that linked a person's past, their current symptoms, and the influence of the therapist. A theory about transference emerged with Strachey translating the German word, übertragung, as 'false connection' (Freud 1894: 301). However, 'false' implies something untrue or wrong, so I translate it as 'mistaken connection', where the person mistakes the therapist for someone from their past but still connects with the therapist. Freud talks about transference in his unsuccessful case of Dora (1905c). In transference, there is an unconscious link made between feelings-states (often unresolved) from the past and the person of the therapist. The therapist does not deserve or create these feelings, they already existed. What the therapist does is create the climate in which the seeds of unconscious material come to life and break through the (conscious) soil above. Often the trigger is some aspect of the therapeutic frame. Through transference, we learn of the relative importance of key figures from the past. The client gets the opportunity to remember and to re-invent what the relationship was like. This may be a recovery, which helps their relationship now. It may be the opportunity to repair damage done early on. It allows the client to take in a new relationship (often called an 'object') that balances out the complexity of positive and negative objects in their internal world.

In subsequent therapy, Terry paid each month by handing me a cheque. One month, he forgot his cheque-book. Another month, he forgot to sign the cheque that he had written earlier and given to me in an envelope. We examined these incidents to see what form of transference was at work. It took us back to his father who gambled (and lost), calculating everything, apart from the emotional impact on his children, which they were now paying for, literally. Terry longed for a father who would simply love him, and part of him resented having to pay me. His fantasy was that he would become special 'like a son', that he would be part of the family and not need to pay.

In transference, when clients hate you, or love you, they feel this with an emotional intensity no matter what goes on in their rational mind. Freud's limited understanding of transference is seen in his treatment of Dora (1905c). He misunderstood the intensity of her transferential feelings that caused her to leave therapy. Having learnt from this transference, Freud later warned therapists (or physicians) about their patients falling in love with them.

Focusing mainly on transference-love and erotic transference

Powerful feelings towards the therapist can be understood as forms of transference-love and erotic transference. Dynamic therapists often encounter transference-love throughout the whole work of therapy, which at times becomes more focused and expressed as erotic transference. Transference-love is, therefore, both general and particular. It takes us back to our very origins and the pulsing desire of every human being expressed in the question, 'Does anyone love me?' or 'Do you love me?' Unless we can answer this, we may as well shut up shop. Freud captured this insight in his early writings where he saw it expressed in our need to remember and repeat our earliest experiences, where the role of the analyst was to understand and interpret thus bringing further insight and change. Later analysts such as Schafer (1977) placed more emphasis on lived encounters infused by the loving presence of the therapist. Schafer writes,

> . . . transference is a piece of real life that is adapted to the analytic purpose, a transitional state of a provisional character this is a means to a rational end and as genuine as normal love. (From this side flows the emphasis in our literature on the healing powers inherent in the therapeutic relationship itself, especially with respect to early privations and deprivations).
>
> (1977: 340)

We heal our client by loving them in an ordinary way, just like Winnicott's ordinary devoted mother (Abram 2013). The work of therapy is to clear the obstacles, overcome the resistances, and help the client let down their defences in order to enable this loving to happen. Our challenge is to enable clients to encounter us as important people who they dare to believe might love them – but not possess them. To love them enough to allow them to become their own person rather than a person shaped in the image of some parental or other significant figure. Clients, too, are muddled about what they want and who they encounter in and through the person of the therapist. Often, they don't know who but they do know what they want: to be loved. Paradoxically, they resist getting close to the therapist, as the fear of intimacy can be too much. Yet if they can, it is enormously beneficial.

Danni's story

Danni is an attractive, vivacious woman doing well in her career. She is stubborn, independent, feisty, and good fun. However, she has problems with intimacy. No man is ever good enough. She goes on dates but at some point the relationship crashes.

Her friend assumed she had 'father' issues; however, therapy helped her see that the problem lay not in an internalised father-figure, as she thought, but instead she had unconsciously assumed the role of her critical mother. When Danni came to therapy, she had taken in the message that only perfection was good enough, an issue re-enforced by her career as a surgeon, where a mistake could prove fatal.

Danni did not find therapy easy, as she felt she was giving up control, though it eventually dawned on her that her therapist was not trying to make her into someone other than herself. Despite Danni's request, the therapist refused to tell her what to do and enabled her to see that when he said that, he really meant it. There was no unspoken code. In therapy, she is learning to be loved and accepted, and trusted to make her own choices. This is a core value in all therapeutic approaches, but a psychodynamic approach deals with what gets in the way, consciously and unconsciously, identified by and worked through in transference phenomena.

Erotic transference

A more focused form of transference-love is expressed as erotic transference, which Freud believed needed to be guarded against (Person and Target 2013). Erotic transference is an important area, and a powerful aspect of dynamic therapy that can be worked with creatively.

Gill's story

Gill loved her therapist, Jake (whom I was supervising). In supervision, when Jake mentioned this he looked terrified, like a rabbit caught in headlights. 'What do I do?', he asked plaintively. As he listened to Gill's story, she told of a cold absent father that she longed to impress and for whom she would do anything. It was clear that all Gill really wanted was to be told by him that she was a lovely girl, the best girl in the world.

Gill's life was littered with broken relationships where she sought to please men who turned out, despite surface appearance, to be emotionally cold and controlling. Jake's emotional warmth and empathic understanding created a powerful intimacy. Jake addressed the idealised and erotic transference (without using those words) and helped Gill to discover that others valued and loved her, too. Often, she discounted their comments, seeking it instead from the one person (her father) who could or would not give it to her.

Realising how she had longed for acceptance as a woman helped Gill see she could change the pattern of her relationships.

Alongside this is the recognition that, if our therapeutic work elicits sexual and/or loving feelings in the therapist (not just the client), these need to be communicated with a clinical supervisor and contained by the therapist. Although there is nothing wrong with erotic feelings, the clinical issue is what they communicate about the therapeutic work. A therapist needs to be able to own their own feelings and, in this way, model to their client that they, too, can accept their powerful sexual and loving feelings. Sadly, there are times when a therapist oversteps the mark and comes to believe their client really does love them or wants to engage with them in a sexual way. To do so is to enter into a boundary violation, representing a lack of professionalism, an ethical lapse, and often repeats early abuse. Yet therapists are human and make mistakes.

Gabbard (2016) has done invaluable work on boundary violations, exploring what lays behind these occurrences. Therapists are vulnerable and some common factors identified were:

- a history of abuse;
- unmet narcissistic needs;
- the need for validation;
- relationship break-up;
- professional isolation; and
- loneliness.

There was also evidence that some therapists enjoyed the abuse of power and were serial offenders until caught. While attending an international conference, I met a new colleague. We enjoyed each other's company and explored who and what we had in common. I mentioned someone, at which point he became silent. It transpired he had referred several clients to this therapist only to discover later that this therapist had gone on to have sexual relationships with them. He was devastated, as he felt his reputation as a therapist was called into question, but more importantly he was left with a gnawing sense of guilt about the impact on the exploited clients. Transference-love and erotic transference are vitally important tools in psychodynamic work and are used to great effect in helping clients discover they are loved.

Transference phenomena are not limited to therapy, although therapy creates a context in which they more readily emerge. The uniqueness of psychodynamic therapies is their encouragement of transference with a therapist who can work with it. No therapist is perfect and we all get transference wrong at some point, though with the right supervision this can enable us to develop as therapists – even through our mistakes (Casement 2002). Transference is ubiquitous and can be found in social groups, work contexts, educational settings, and the like. It is triggered by some aspect of the other person, such as the way they look, sound, respond, even a mannerism that triggers unconscious feelings.

A student's story

While teaching psychodynamic theory (on an integrative course), there was one student who always looked disengaged. When she did engage, it was in an argumentative, hostile manner saying, 'Why do we need to learn about Freud anyway? He's so out of date'. She would avoid any groups I facilitated until the second year when she had no choice.

In a session on 'working with abuse', I disclosed a personal experience. Sometime later, she asked to see me and told me she was sorry for the way she had been acting. Bravely, she disclosed that an older family member, who had a grey beard and soft Scottish accent like mine, had abused her. She experienced me as a harsh tutor who was telling her she was not good enough as a student, neither of which was true. So an aspect of me triggered a transference response as if I were an abusing uncle she was powerless to defend herself from. That was why she tried to keep me away through her verbal barbs, which satisfied her angry feelings. What changed was my disclosure, as she realised that I was not the awful figure I had become in her fantasy. It also modelled to her that if I, as some form of authority figure, could be open about an abusive experience, so could she.

Through transference, we learn of the relative importance of key figures from the past. The client gets the opportunity to remember what the relationship was like. This may be a recovery, which helps their relationship now. It may be the opportunity to repair damage done early on. Either way, it allows the client to take in a new relationship that balances out the complexity of positive and negative objects in their internal world.

Focusing mainly on counter-transference

Nowadays, it is almost impossible to separate transference and counter-transference, both fitting together like hand and glove. Counter-transference emerged in the 1950s, marking a watershed in psychodynamic clinical practice (Stefana 2017). In 1947, Winnicott initiated this with a complex paper, *Hate in the Counter-transference*, where he encourages the therapist to experience and express their love and hate for the client (Caldwell and Joyce 2011). When I was a trainee and introduced to this idea for the first time, I was shocked. How could a therapist wanting to help a client hate them but, possibly even worse, let the client know? Winnicott, in his ironic and playful use of words, gets to a core issue of what the therapist feels in and through their counter-transference and how this becomes a central feature of their work. As therapists, if we avoid the depth of our feelings, we end up splitting (Chapter 5) and fail to model a different way of being for our clients. After all, mothers both love and hate their babies. The sheer demands of the newborn, their state of utter helplessness recalling our utter helplessness, the radical change a baby brings to a person's life including joy and loss, echo back through time and reverberate around the unconscious. A similar vortex of feelings and thoughts arise when encountering our clients.

Infant development and neuroscience have enabled us to see minute interactions that communicate profound internal states between the client and therapist, and as such provide a solid foundation for psychological growth, if all goes well. If the therapist is able to repeat such minute interactions, it enables the client to tolerate gaps, mistakes, and ruptures, and allows them to give up the idealised figure of their fantasy for the ordinariness of the therapist where they, too, can be human.

Embodied counter-transference

How client and therapist reach this point can be found in and through the use of counter-transference, especially in its somatic, bodily-based expressions. Where we encounter unconscious material drawn from the client's pre-verbal stage of development, or from early trauma and dissociation, we are more likely to discover this in our body than anywhere else. By listening to our body, we can reach the minds of our clients (Blechner 2011), enhance the quality of our interpretations, and enable new and living connections for our clients

(Field 1989). One common form of embodied counter-transference is feeling tired or falling asleep when with a client.

Dace's story

I saw Dace for six sessions in a university counselling service. We had little control over the heating in the room, which was often stuffy. At first, I thought it was just that, but when I felt I was nodding off in weeks two and three, it dawned on me that something was happening out of my conscious awareness. On the surface, Dace seemed to be coping with the prospect of an arranged marriage but found it more and more difficult to focus on her work for her final exams. Supervision helped me see that my starting to fall asleep was an embodied defence against going anywhere near the core issues of rage and depression.

Subsequent experience has told me this is a common defence of mine, which I can also encounter when working with therapists in supervision where they are working with clients hiding their anger or rage. Understanding and using counter-transference is a vital skill in dynamic therapies as long as we are able to distinguish what belongs to us from what belongs to the client. It is always important to remind ourselves that in any counter-transference response, there is the possibility this contains aspects of the therapist's transference to the client.

Having examined some of the complexities concerning transference and counter-transference as a trainee or newly qualified therapist, I would be wondering how to make sense of it all. Lacan offers some uncharacteristically simple wisdom that de-mystifies transference when he writes, 'positive transference is when you have a soft spot for the individual concerned . . . and the negative transference is when you have to keep an eye on him' (1977: 124), and I would add 'as well as ourselves'.

Using supervision creatively

Over the years, I have supervised many trainees and experienced therapists, including some from the integrative tradition who want to incorporate psychodynamic ways of working in their practice. The therapists I have enjoyed most working with are those who see supervision as a creative, exploratory space where they can risk talking about their mistakes and are open to different ways of thinking and feeling (Webb and Wheeler 1998). This is where supervision proves especially important (Wheeler and Richards 2007) and why psychodynamic supervision is essential for the on-going growth in knowledge and experience of the therapist (Howard 2017).

Jenny's story

Jenny came back to see me after completing her four-year psychodynamic training. Professionally accredited and employed as a therapist, she worked with the supervisor provided by the agency who was from an integrative background. While Jenny found this helpful, she discovered to her surprise that she missed the rigour of supervision from her psychodynamic training. With fear and trepidation, Jenny approached me to see if I would be willing to supervise her again.

In the first session, we explored how she used to experience me as a critical tutor. We unpacked that I was not critical; this was something from a past transference, and we examined what the differences might be. Moving from a tutor–student relationship to a collegial relationship is always challenging but it is such a joy as a trainer to see a new generation of therapists grow into their therapeutic potential.

The psychodynamic processes we have examined, relating to the therapist and client, can be replicated in the supervisory relationship. Just as in therapy, supervision for a therapist should be the place they come alive to their therapeutic work. At its best, it is a place of trust and creativity. Just as in good therapy, this requires developing a creative alliance with the supervisor, a feature found across all therapeutic modalities (Bambling et al. 2006). Once established, this enables a supervisee to explore the mistakes, clarify their confusions, think differently, discover their and their clients' projections, untangle transferences and counter-transferences, and re-work triangular relationships. Supervision enables us to address issues of social and cultural difference and diversity that inevitably arise in our work (Watkins 2016), as well as being a vital place for ethical discussion and reflection, whether clinical- or research-related (Danchev and Ross 2013).

In the course of this book, we have moved from a one-person psychoanalytic approach (Freud), through a two-person approach (object-relations – Klein, Bion, Winnicott, Kohut, Bollas), to arrive at a relational psychoanalytic perspective focused on co-created intersubjectivity. These changes have been captured by the fixed, rugged, and dancing landscape model, and influence the way we experience supervision. My early supervision located me as a novice and my supervisor as the expert. My next supervision was still in this vein but drew on broader Freudian and Jungian perspectives. My most creative experience of supervision has been a co-creative encounter working with what was happening in the room, between my clients and me and my supervisor (Frawley-O'Dea and Sarnat 2001). So supervision works best as a collegial relationship and, as the supervisor, I find supervisees engaging to work with because they always have something to teach me. When I encourage supervisees to bring their whole person into the supervisory space, I'm also clear it is not a substitute for therapy.

Nick's story

Nick was a qualified psychodynamic therapist who had been practising for a couple of years. His previous supervisor was retiring and so he met with me as a possible replacement. Nick was thoughtful, open, willing to learn, and in many respects a potentially good supervisee. But despite doing well professionally, it became clear his personal life was in carnage. Estranged from his partner, Nick felt very isolated, and my increasing anxiety was that he was living his life through his work.

We arranged two sessions of supervision (during which I had my own supervision), at which point I suggested that we needed to stop. Nick was talking more and more about himself and less and less about his clients. I explored whether he needed to return to his own therapy. He was resistant to hear this as he felt he had 'done' therapy and what was happening in his personal life was just temporary. I disagreed and we had a difficult ending. I never did find out what happened next.

Working with resistance

Having engaged with the beating heart of psychodynamic therapies, it is helpful now to turn to resistance, the iron-will that is conscious, but most often unconscious, that tries to block progress at every turn.

Freud highlighted the importance of resistance in *Remembering, Repeating and Working-Through* (1914b). In the Second World War, the French Resistance emerged to oppose the German occupying powers. The title of Gildea's gripping history of the Resistance, *Fighters in the Shadows* (2015), captures the forms of psychological resistance we encounter with our clients. They are not immediately obvious, with a shadow-like existence, but all too powerful in action.

Historically, identifying and working to overcome a client's resistance about conscious fears and fantasies formed a central part of analytic work and shaped interpretations. Directly challenging a client when they deny something can be like running into a brick wall. Defences are an important way we keep our core or true self safe in the past, and so must be respected. In my experience, every client comes to therapy with a desire to change and a desire to stay the same. Change is difficult or, as one client said, 'What happens if I don't like the new me?'

Another reason clients come to therapy is because they have developed such a strong attachment to a figure or object-relation in their internal world, it has become pathological. Consider the following vignette.

Shona's story

Shona has done amazingly well in her career and is widely liked and respected. Nobody has a bad word to say about her, apart from the men she has relationships with. It was because of relationship issues she came for therapy. Shona talked about her idyllic childhood dominated by her father and brother. She discovered that men leave her because in her psyche she has an image of the perfect man, modelled on her father and brothers. Nobody ever comes up to scratch; they leave because they cannot compete.

It haunts the psyche, but is elusive, generating the thought that they can never imagine being free. Like an addict, giving up what is killing them is hard to do, as Freud discovered in his passion for cigars (Ross 2016b). Yet avoiding challenging this pathological attachment becomes a form of collusion to avoid disturbing the status quo, and very often such a dynamic pull in us is a direct repeat of an early family pattern, 'Don't upset your father/mother'. A feature of an intersubjective approach to resistance when it emerges also has to do with the resistance in the therapist. Maybe we, too, have difficulty in facing that early familial pattern.

Facing and accepting endings

After three years of therapy (lying on a couch twice a week), I decided it was time to finish. It was not a sudden flash of insight, rather a growing awareness that, valuable as therapy was, it was also possible *not* to be in therapy. It was a recognition that I could decide even about something I did not find easy, as I have always hated endings. (The story of my life has been one of premature arrivals and abrupt endings.) It took nine months to end, as my therapist and I worked through aspects that we could not have done if the therapy had been on-going. It was a good-enough ending and a personal reminder that, in psychodynamic work, there is something distinctive about the end of therapy (Murdin 2015). Sometimes it is planned, often unplanned, and occasionally unilateral when a client just stops coming.

My daughter's story

My daughter rang up and said, 'Dad, how do you sack a therapist? I've got a session coming up later today and I've decided my therapist's not challenging enough. He's very nice but I think I want more'. I suggested that she should talk to him in the next session and mention she was thinking of leaving and then arrange at least one session (they had six already) where they both knew exactly what was on the agenda. I did point out that, as a psychodynamic therapist, I would normally want to work towards an ending that was shared. They had one final session and she made what appeared to be a good ending, although I have no idea what this therapist made of this or talked about with his supervisor.

We all face endings. Therapist and client circumstances take over, life-events happen, money runs out, partners leave, illness intervenes, death strikes, employment relocates us, and looming and unwanted retirement beckons. Endings take on an even greater importance in time-limited therapy. The rule of thumb is that you work with the ending from the very beginning. Precisely because endings are so powerful, and can be so damaging if handled badly, they need a clear focus. In any therapeutic work, we never know what we will encounter. Yet we can be certain of one thing: any client will have an untold history of loss and endings.

Therapy is an opportunity to take control of an ending, to re-shape or re-work a prior ending, to acknowledge the pain or sadness of previous losses. No ending is ever complete. There are always untimely moments, incomplete conversations, unspoken thoughts and feelings, that touch on areas deep within us of love, hate, pain, and hope – usually a combination of them all. Everyone has mixed feelings about endings and so there is often a level of ambivalence, like growing up where we want to be the adult, but we want to retain those childish or child-like experiences. This is a normal part of being human. As a child, some experiences were so exciting, so all-consuming that we wished they would never come to an end and, in a moment of magical thinking, believed they would go on forever. Such a fantasy is built on the symbiotic oneness of our earliest experiences where the body, mind, self, and psyche merge into one ultimate sense of bliss. In the absence of this bliss, or the taking away of bliss, the results can be an un-verbalised, symbolised experience of utter desolation and primal rage. The unconscious, among other things, is a repository, a psychic waiting room for the last train out of town.

Every ending is like a death in miniature. I do not wish to be disrespectful to the 'guts ripped out of you' experience of losing someone close to you. We live in a society that finds it difficult to deal with grief, so it is all the more important in therapy that endings work on issues of loss and grief, as well as recapturing the richness and learning the client has worked towards. In the sixteen-session brief model used in DIT (Lemma et al. 2011), there is the opportunity to capture what had gone on in the therapy by a 'goodbye' letter. This captures what the work has been about, what the client has learnt, what resources they have discovered, and what they may need to continue to work on. Such letters are challenging to write but profoundly helpful.

Rachel's story

I was close to finishing my sixteen sessions with Rachel, an archaeology student, when they came to an abrupt ending following my fall down a mountain (Ross 2014, 2016a). I was off work for six months and so she continued her therapy with a colleague. There was something left unfinished between us, so on my return, I arranged to see her for a final session. Rachel readily agreed, recognising that we could both acknowledge an appropriate ending, disrupted as this was.

The paradox was that her life history was of people leaving her and having to fend for herself. At the age of nine, her father departed, leaving her with an alcoholic mother to care for. In our final session, Rachel expressed relief that we had both survived our very different life-threatening experiences and what we did was 'good-enough', a phrase she proudly told me she had learned from Winnicott. I was profoundly touched. Sometimes the therapy is good for the therapist as well as the client.

The business of therapy

Many therapists work in private practice, a trend that is increasing as cognitive-based therapies are coming to dominate the NHS to the exclusion of other therapeutic traditions. Given that psychodynamic therapists often work with clients over a longer period of time, in the financially stretched NHS where cost-cutting is rife, they are increasingly an endangered species. It is important therefore to pay attention to the details of how therapy works as a business, whether in private practice or in voluntary contexts (Hodson 2012).

Here is a brief overview of what therapists need to consider in setting out a contract to work professionally and ethically (Mitchels and Bond 2011). Clients need to know what it is they are signing up to because if they have never had therapy before, they cannot know what to expect. A clear, simple contract (verbal and written) outlines important details that give the client the information they need to consent to therapy.

Expectations

Clients often ask, 'will therapy help me or solve my problems?' I explain that people come with a presenting problem, which may or may not be the issue we work on together. I explain that psychodynamic therapists work with the influence of the past on the present, and with the emergence of unconscious processes, so we never quite know what will happen. This is helpful to discuss in an initial session because it clarifies what they expect, which while often realistic, can identify issues that may be unrealistic (see Julia earlier in the chapter).

Following a car accident, I was seeing a physiotherapist who explained that she could only help the affected joints recover to the level of function they had before the accident. She could not repair any damage that pre-existed the accident. Similarly, I can say to clients that they will gain insight, make connections, discover meaning, and have someone who will not judge – but they will be re-visiting scenes from the past. This process can often lead to symptom reduction but, as in all psychodynamic therapies, this is their *raison d'être*.

Timings and duration

Psychodynamic therapists normally work in 50-minute sessions, at the same time and day, on a weekly or more frequent basis. Clients need to know what to do with breaks to this pattern caused by holiday or illness. Do they pay for missed or cancelled sessions? One therapist I saw was clear from the outset that I was expected to pay for our two sessions every week (whether I attended or not).

Clients often ask, 'how long it will take?' I reply that it depends, but we can do six sessions and then review if they want to move to an open-ended basis. I say that, if they were to give one session for every year of their life, we could be here for thirty, forty, or fifty sessions. Clients really get this. Terry (earlier in this chapter) wanted six sessions but stayed for two years as he realised in that first six sessions the depth of issues on which he needed to work. We only stopped then because I was moving out of London.

Boundaries

It is important that clients understand the limitations of therapy, the therapeutic relationship, and the importance of boundaries. Some clients new to therapy want to make you their friend. A client might want to contact you between sessions. While all therapists can be friendly, respectful, and interested in their clients, it is the nature of a boundaried relationship that enables therapy to work. For example, a psychodynamic therapist should decline a client's request to be friends on social media. It is always important to keep in mind what psychodynamic processes are being played out.

Other important, ethical boundaries in therapy include refraining from sexual, financial, or psychological exploitation of one's clients, though sadly exploitation happens (Gabbard 2016). As we saw in Chapter 12, one of the toxic legacies of sexual abuse or grooming is that the clients no longer know where boundaries are, not so much intellectually but *emotionally*. We need boundaries throughout our life to help us understand who we are, where we belong, and how we fit with others.

Confidentiality

If a client asks, 'Is therapy absolutely confidential?', the answer needs to be 'no'. This gives the therapist the opportunity to clarify the limits of confidentiality.

- First, there are a number of legal requirements, such as if a client tells you they are the member or a supporter of a terrorist organisation (this has happened to me once).

- Second, where there is a risk of harm to the client or others, you may need to refer the client for specialist help. Camilla was on anti-depressant medication but her suicidal feelings had increased. I was sufficiently concerned and suggested to her that it might be helpful for me to talk with her GP (who she was seeing regularly). Camilla agreed to this but, if she had not, I would have still contacted her GP as I believed her suicidal thoughts were severe and that she may not have been telling her GP the whole truth. I believed that she was a serious risk but was also trying to maintain a therapeutic relationship that could survive me taking this action.

- Third, there should be the on-going expectation of discussing client work with a supervisor, though I assure clients that even here the work is anonymised as much as possible.

- Fourth, in a training or placement context, there is group rather than an individual confidentiality.

Wherever possible, even if I believe there is a need to break confidentiality, I would try to discuss this with a client as the strength of the therapeutic relationship may be able to survive this breach. Confidentiality is complicated and not always clear-cut. It raises ethical dilemmas, which need to be discussed in supervision or with someone with suitable expertise. For example, in working with refugees and trafficked women, reporting an issue may put them at even greater risk.

Contact and communication

Clients most commonly approach us using email, telephone, or text. When meeting for an assessment, the therapist records contact details such as: address; telephone; email; and their GP's name, address, and contact details. It is important to ask how they wish to be contacted, if necessary.

After each session, most therapists keep brief notes, which are kept securely on a password-encrypted computer or in a locked container. This means that therapists need to register as 'controllers' in order to meet the requirements of the General Data Protection Regulation (GDPR) by the Information Commissioner's Office, an independent authority established to protect personal data. Having registered, therapists need to have a transparent process that allows clients to see any data they hold on them in any form and how they protect this. As a psychodynamic therapist, if a client asks to see their notes, it would be important to work with them to discern why they are requesting this and examine what might be going on at a therapeutic level. It is equally important, however, to give the access they have requested.

I keep paper records, including copies of emails that I print out then delete from my computer. These records are shredded after seven years. (In the case of Megan [Chapter 8], who asked to hold her photograph, if she had not required this within the seven years, I would have returned this to her.)

Finances

Clients ask, 'how much it will cost?' This is an entirely reasonable and commonplace request. If a dent on my car needs fixing, I ask how much it will cost to fix. If I am asked to speak at a conference, I am asked how much I charge, or I am told 'we would like you to speak and this is the fee we offer'. Some therapists have a fixed fee, while others operate a sliding scale.

In the past, I have benefitted from a therapist offering me reduced fees, as that was all I could afford. Some therapists adjust their fees depending on the client's circumstances. It is important to note, however, that just because a client is paying a reduced fee, it does not make them any less demanding to work with. It is also helpful to know when and how the client will pay for the therapy. Some pay every session. Most pay by bank transfer on a sessional or monthly basis.

Janet's story

Janet was in her twenties and came to see me because her marriage had broken down, leaving her with large debts. I queried whether she could afford counselling, even at the reduced rate I was offering. Janet said that she could not afford to make another mistake in relationships and so it was money well spent. She paid every session in cash because 'it is real money', unlike the thousands of pounds of debt she had built up on her credit card.

Therapists also need to keep records of their income and costs in the form of simple accounts that can be used for tax purposes and available for audit (if required). As your private practice grows, it may be advisable to employ an accountant.

Advertising

Clients do not just turn up on your doorstep demanding to be seen. The success of any private practice is linked to the range of referral networks to which you have access. It is this entrepreneurial dimension that stops some therapists from making the transition to private practice. Many who do choose to advertise on various websites specifically designed for clients looking for therapists. People often ask me if I know a therapist I can recommend in a certain area. Often I do, but if I don't I look at the same websites; the difference is that I know what I am looking for. Every time I do this, I am shocked by the wide-ranging claims many therapists make. Integrative therapists can legitimately offer therapy across a range of modalities, but psychodynamic therapists would be moving beyond the parameters of their training if they did so.

Ethically, it is good to advertise what you can do from a psychodynamic perspective and who you can work with, trusting that the right clients will find you. For example, I am not a trained couples' therapist, but very occasionally I will do a one-off consultation to help a couple decide what they want to do as part of a process of referring them on to colleagues. I am happy to see an individual who may also be in couples' therapy, however. In contrast, many individually trained therapists claim on their website that they can see couples. It is best to advertise who we are and what we do, confident in our training and our level of expertise. This is in line with a wider ethical commitment to integrity, transparency, and working in the best interests of the client.

Thinking and working ethically

Therapists are often uncomfortable around the subject of ethics, thinking it is either an intellectual juggling act full of impossible scenarios with no clear-cut and definitive answers, or some form of covert police trying to catch us out.

The place to begin is to realise that ethics is about the kind of person you want to be. It relates directly to who you are, not just what you do or decide as a therapist. Our ethics hold our most important values and beliefs about life, meaning, and well-being for ourselves and for the other (Proctor 2014). Every professional body has an ethical code or framework that is often filed on the bookshelf for 'rarely read books and documents too important to throw away' or stored in a little-visited part of the computer's hard-drive. Best practice would be for you to talk regularly with a supervisor about an ethical review of your work, not just in a crisis over confidentiality or some other matter about boundaries (Amis 2017). Historically, psychoanalytic and psychodynamic thinking has neglected ethics, although Freud had a great deal to say about individual and collective values that stimulates new debates around ethics (Wallwork 2012). One contemporary psychodynamic approach sees the emergence of relational ethics, as informed by four strands:

- professional standard codes of ethical practice;
- our particular dynamic theoretical orientation, which involves the known and the unknown;
- our personal ethics, including truth, honesty, fluidity, spirituality, and our view of the other; and
- communal ethics, our connection to something other than the individual, including the group and the society (Barsness and Strawn 2018).

Summary

The foundation skills we have explored in this chapter are about transforming theory into practice, motivated by love for another human being. Here, love is a longing for the other to be whole.

It has taken us real graft and lungfuls of oxygen to get here, not by the most direct route but by following the curve of a ridge shaped in volcanic times in order to reach the summit – the unconscious. The views are glorious, just like the unique psyche of each living, breathing client we see. We started with assessment and formulation – easy to say, less easy to do. We then developed a therapeutic alliance – building an empathy that opens the depths of another. We then understood the role of complex past relationships (part and whole), using transference and counter-transference – this required us to work with resistance, and there is often resistance around endings, painful as these are for clients and therapists.

With the growth of private practice for psychodynamic therapists, it is important that we attend to the business of being a therapist. The next chapter explores new skills we can add to these essential foundations.

Reflective questions

Which of these foundational skills do you find the most challenging?

What issues does this raise for you that you could take to supervision or study further?

What aspect of the business of therapists may need further attention?

If applicable, when will you book in with your supervisor for an ethical review?

Looking at research

Research on competencies that underpin the skills outlined can be found in Lemma, Roth and Pilling (2008) *The Competencies Required to Deliver Effective Psychoanalytic/ Psychodynamic Therapy* and UCL's online guide to Psychoanalytic/Psychodynamic Therapy, available at:

https://www.ucl.ac.uk/pals/research/clinical-educational-and-health-psychology/ research-groups/core/competence-frameworks-6 [accessed 16 October 2018].

Similarly, there are further competencies for supervision (not just psychodynamic) by Tony Roth and Stephen Pilling (developed and revised 2007/2015) and UCL's online guide to Supervision of Psychological Therapies, available at:

https://www.ucl.ac.uk/pals/research/clinical-educational-and-health-psychology/ research-groups/core/competence-frameworks-8 [accessed 16 October 2018].

14

Developing skills for practice

There are a number of important psychodynamic skills that it takes time and experience to get the hang of. I would love to say we can master these but this implies we can reach that elusive stage. We are always learning and every new client is a fresh opportunity to engage with another's psyche at depth and with all the attendant dynamics we have looked at throughout this book. Yet there is another danger: not that we become too confident, but that we don't become confident enough. We can set ourselves such high goals (often influenced by an overly active super-ego) that we always feel we have failed or never done enough. The following skills reach further into us and our clients in ways that enhance our psychodynamic practice.

Assessment re-visited

In counselling agencies (professional or voluntary), it is essential to have the most experienced therapists doing assessments. This is especially important for trainees who do not yet have the experience to deal with co-morbid clients with long-standing health and mental health issues, suicidal ideation, self-harm, acting out, or other risk behaviours. These are complex clinical cases with clients who have multiple needs.

In my experience, over thirty years as a therapist, the level of need in clients and the severity of the problems or issues that clients bring has increased exponentially. Therefore, the need to match the right client with the right therapist is vital. For therapists in private practice, this is an especially important area to focus on because, other than support through clinical supervision or colleagues, the buck stops with you.

Dynamic seeing

There is a further skill we can develop at the assessment stage – *seeing the future*. Therapists are not clairvoyants and do not have any secret knowledge. They do, however, have an ability to imagine what the client might become beyond problem-solving or symptom reduction. We can imagine trying to see into the future if the client has the resources for any exploration of the unconscious. We ask the questions, 'What can I "see" in this client?' Can I "see" beyond what they see or want at some unspoken level?' What did I see in Terry (Chapter 13)? I saw ghosts from the past that were haunting him in the present – they were waiting in his unconscious for resurrection. In Terry, I 'saw' that once these ethereal bit-part actors had been heard on stage, they could depart and leave him in peace.

Alex Danchev, writing about a British military historian, gives an insight into the man:

> What he dreamed, what he dreaded, what he detested, what he desired – the ghosts that drove him – these are the things that hook us in.
>
> (1998: 5)

In our unconscious state, we are

> a blend of brooding dread and somnambulistic eroticism, passive, bewitched, yet also seeking, among the wreckage of the outer and inner worlds in which we were astray . . . some pearl beyond price just behind and beyond the veil.
>
> (Raine quoted in Danchev 1998: 11)

Danchev unknowingly captures the essence of psychodynamic therapy. It is all about our dreams, dreads, dislikes, and desires.

Contemporary psychodynamic therapy adds the concept of 'dynamic seeing'. Imagine the profound gaze of a mother and a baby. Infant research tells us how vital this is for the psychical foundations and subsequent well-being of the baby. A mother, father, or caregiver hold and look at a little, helpless, wriggling bundle of life and see into the future. Already they are holding the baby in mind as a person, not a thing, and not yet formed, just in the process of becoming. At the assessment stage, we see beyond the presenting problem, the story of the client's past, the traumas touched on, and the transferential hints we pick up. We can 'see' into the unconscious of the client by attending to the images that appear in our mind, which may tell us what lies ahead. My 'dynamic seeing' of a client at assessment is a visual picture of the unconscious in their inner world, populated by internal objects. What I see are similar to the biomorphic forms sculpted by Henry Moore or Barbara Hepworth against an ink-black starry sky. They move in and out of focus. With Terry, the experience was profound as all I could see was one far-distant object on which I could barely focus. This told me, and subsequent therapy proved, that he was hard to reach, terrified of losing the one good internal object he possessed, but hungry for more.

Working with projective identification

First elaborated by Klein, projective identification is where the client unconsciously projects their unwanted feelings onto the therapist, who begins to identify with them. A client may seem unusually calm while describing a dreadful situation, but the therapist feels overwhelming anger for no rational reason. The client's unwanted rage has been communicated in such a way as to be experienced by the therapist in much the same way a baby communicates powerful feelings in a mother without words.

Projective processes

Klein's distinctive views of the timing of transference and focus on projective identification is captured in Ogden (1992) and Spillius and O'Shaughnessy (2012). Klein understood transference, counter-transference, and projective processes as a framework containing all dynamic processes, which Joseph (1985) describes as a 'total situation'. Likewise, Ogden (1986) believes it is impossible to understand any transference process without using projective identification, processes that Finlay describes as 'fascinating, mysterious, slippery, and seductive' (2016: 202). Such a description leaves me wanting to know more. In reality, there is a particular quality to experiencing the power of a projective experience that marks it out.

So what is happening when we say something is projective identification? There are four aspects, all unconscious.

- First, it is a way of letting the therapist know that something is important by getting into the psyche of the other person.

- Second, it is a useful way of getting rid of the unwanted thoughts and feelings of one's psyche by emptying them in the skip of another's mind, hopefully to be taken away.

- Third, it acts like some form of primitive mother–baby fusion where there is no separation, thus replaying an early maternal relationship.

- Fourth, and less commonly, in some contexts a client feels safe enough to project an aspect of himself or herself, or a dissociative state or person, which the therapist catches sight of and invites into the therapy. We can identify it through Winnicott's me-not-me process. We are sitting with a client and then feel or say something that makes us think, 'Where did that come from? Was that really me?'. In that moment, we have acted into the role projected into us or acted out the feelings projected into us as if we were the client. This me-not-me idea becomes even more important in varying forms of intersubjective connection.

Intersubjective connections

Intersubjective connection is a form of relatedness that occurs when the client and therapist bring their subjectivities into the room. It is a psychological co-creation with conscious and unconscious dimensions. We can understand this by appreciating that therapy is an all too human encounter, one in which we are moved, touched, angered, frustrated with our clients, and they us in a reciprocal, interpersonal dance. The steps are both remembered from the past and alive in the moment.

Annabelle's story

Annabelle came into the room looking enormously sad. Her pain-wracked face, bleary eyes, absence of make-up (an unusual occurrence), and faintly mismatched and dishevelled clothing told me something was badly wrong. 'He's left me', she said and became silent. The silence stretched on until, out of this space of unspoken grief, she declared, 'After all this time in therapy thinking about how bad my relationship with Jim was, now he's gone, I still love him'.

The distraught nature of her sadness was palpable and I, too, felt a crushing sense of loss, both in the room containing our shared therapy space and in me as I recalled some of my own losses. From a traditional psychodynamic perspective, it would be inappropriate for me to talk about my loss, as I would be imposing my needs or agenda on the client. From an intersubjective perspective, it may be appropriate, depending on the co-created intersubjective encounter present in the clinical work, which varies from client to client.

My response to Annabelle was to wait, silently letting the ever-present unconscious communicate to her there was something shared in this space.

Interpersonal and inter-psychic processes occur in the intersubjective space created between therapist and client. This includes what both think and feel about each other, working with resistance, elements of challenge, confrontation, empathy, and exploration. These capture the unique person of the client and that of the therapist. These processes express concern and compassion, depth and insight from both subjectivities. A client needs to believe they matter to us and, while not meeting our needs, they give to us something profound in every session.

My and Izzy's story

After a serious accident, I was unable to do clinical work for six months. I had already taken a break with a client before my accident but had texted to cancel the date we were due to resume when I was still in recovery.

The door-bell went and my wife answered the door to find my 17-year-old client, Izzy, standing there. She had not received my text and had been driven to the session by a parent who was calling back for her in an hour. So Izzy came into the room where I was propped up on a settee (not my normal consulting room). She gasped with horror when she saw me and looked like she was going to cry. Admittedly, it must have been shocking to see me with both legs and one arm in plaster, and a bandaged head. Izzy radiated compassion, not so much in what she said but more through her very being expressed in her body language and eye contact. I realised that I mattered to her far more deeply than I could have known, and she mattered to me.

When we resumed therapy, she told me I looked so bad, she thought I was going to die. Yet, in our intersubjective encounter, she was also telling me she was feeling so bad, *she* wanted to die. We compared the scars on our wrists and acknowledged a shared flirting with death in a way that allowed us to meet in a new way.

Intersubjective processes energise the client in the difficult work of therapy where uncomfortable issues, thoughts, and feelings need to be engaged with. Benjamin (2004) and Ogden (1994) use the term 'the analytic third' to describe this creative process, although they understand this in different ways. This phrase captures something unique that is happening, a new space, form of reflection, and place for insight that makes the therapist and client come alive. Intersubjective transferential processes are: developmental, neurological, pre-natal, mindful, and technical in allowing the unconscious to be the unconscious at work simultaneously in both client and therapist.

Dynamic therapists can thus learn through their clients. What we learn is how we habitually respond in terms of seeing transference in the client, how we draw attention to this, how we use it to shape an interpretation, and how and where we locate counter-transference in us as therapists. Joseph (1985) makes the important point that clients hear or understand our interpretations differently depending on where they are located in their current therapy. Someone in a paranoid-schizoid position, for example, is likely to defend themselves through splitting and using projective identification (unconscious as they are), less likely to hear what is being said, and less able to enter into intersubjective processes.

The phenomenology of transference processes – the way they appear to consciousness – includes projective identification as a more focused aspect of counter-transference. Such phenomena engage us as therapists in a living relationship with constant movement from the past to the present, the present to the past, in and through the therapeutic encounter. The coming together of intersubjectivities allows something new to be created. It is helpful to remember that clients repeat transference, counter-transference, and projective and intersubjective processes through the therapy, and the longer the therapy, the more opportunities there are for this to occur. Like the Post-Impressionist painter Cezanne, who was never happy until he saw on the canvas what appeared in his mind (Danchev 2012), clients become artists who re-work the canvas of their lives through these interweaving transference processes.

Dreaming dreams; working with metaphors

In the immortal words of my colleague Sarah (who was warning her staff at the time), 'Don't sit next to Alistair. Before you know it, you'll be telling him your dreams and discovering stuff you didn't want to know'.

Dreams fascinate and confuse in equal measure. They appeal far beyond the therapeutic discipline. Macbeth, afflicted by no longer being able to sleep, was unable to deal with his traumas through dreaming. Would Lady Macbeth have killed herself had she not been haunted by her dream-like nocturnal vision of bloodied hands? Freud located the origins of psychoanalysis through his own dreams, and *The Interpretation of Dreams* (1900) has had a wide-ranging influence touching many other academic disciplines (Fonagy et al. 2012). In summary, Freud's patients told him dreams, which he would interpret, and lives were thereby changed.

Jung, once the crown prince, heir to the throne, and chosen successor to Freud, was similarly enamoured by the power of dreams and their route to the unconscious, yet time and fashions change. No longer do dynamic therapies wedded to dreams play such a crucial role, and dreams, once regarded as a separate subject worth discussing, have been subsumed under the umbrella of unconscious communication (Howard 2017). This represents a significant and apparently unmourned loss. In part, this is the result of a shift to time-limited therapies with the omnipresent tick-tock of the clock and no space to explore the complexities of dreaming (Hobson 2016). Remember Kat from Chapter 7? It was a dream that enabled her to enter into therapy at a new depth.

Freud believed that in dreams, what is less important is the *content* and what is most important is the dream as a *form of thinking*. Dreams tell us something important about the working of the psyche, but this can be difficult to discern as they often contain powerful images and depths of emotion. In Jungian terms, it is the *relationship* rather than the *interpretation* that is vital, as the dream triggers archaic and archetypal content that can then be explored. The focus is on the texture of the dream as it is being replayed in relationship in therapy. Psychodynamic therapists working with dreams often draw on both Freud and Jung's understandings (see Figure 14.1).

Later analysts developed their dream-work in new ways (see Figure 14.2 for comparison). Grotstein, who had been in analysis with Bion, viewed dreams as telling us about the powerful presences within us, viz. aspects of the self from multiple perspectives, as while there is a person who dreams the dream, what they dream is another person (or themselves) dreaming the dream (2007). So, if my dream were captured on film, it would reveal me imagining myself experiencing a dream. Ogden (1986) introduces the idea of a 'dream space', like a psychic transitional or potential space, that allows something unique to develop by engaging dialectically with an analytic space held by the therapist. Bollas (1987), meanwhile, saw dreams as aesthetic creations that identify unique patterns or idioms.

Dreams reveal to the person something about themselves they need to know, but don't yet know. This approach fits with intersubjective perspectives where dreams cannot be

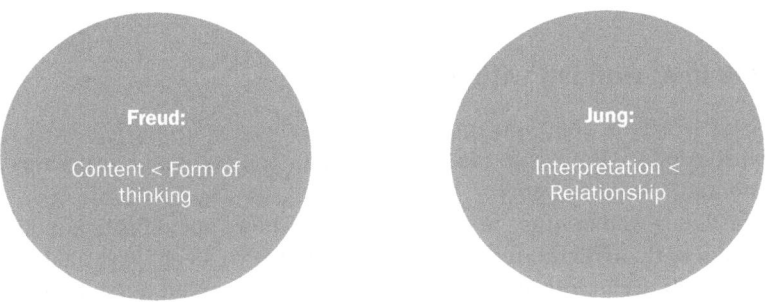

Figure 14.1 Traditional hierarchies of a dream

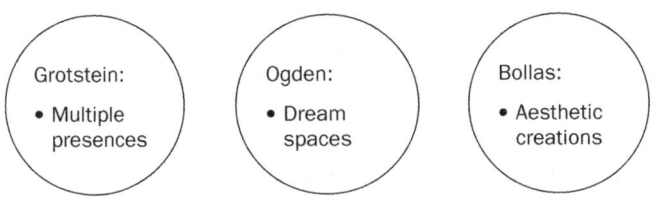

Figure 14.2 Contemporary hierarchies of a dream

understood outside the therapeutic context in which they occur. Yet there is another associated development. We live in a media-saturated, image-rich world that creates the illusion nothing is more than a click away. It is a highly visual culture where there is an increased use of visual metaphors to communicate emotional truths.

Ewan's story

Ewan talked about his collection of action comics and graphic novels. I asked him whom he most identified with. He looked stunned and said, 'Nobody's ever asked me that before. The thought's never crossed my mind'. He had always thought it was just a form of escapism. We worked with this metaphor of 'escape' and how his heroes escaped the original trauma that gave them superpowers. In time, we looked at the hidden traumas that had remained present but unconscious until then in Ewan's life.

Our clients' metaphors (Long and Lepper 2008; Finlay 2016) offer a valuable way of accessing their unconscious associations in the way dreams once did, and indeed still do if time and space permit. This is especially important when working with clients who have experienced early trauma (Leonoff 2013).

There are several ways we can work with dreams and metaphors.

1. Separate manifest and latent content in your mind.
   - The surface connections have one layer of meaning, the hidden connections another, but both are important.
2. Help the client to 'free associate'.
   - This has been taken up far less in psychodynamic counselling and integrative therapies but is still of great value at the right time (Bollas 2007).
3. Recognise that every component of the dream refers to some aspect of the client's life.
4. Ask the client what they make of their dream.
5. Focus on the feelings within the dream, and so identify the very texture of the experience.
6. Reflect on why this dream and why now.
   - The client's dream could be a way of avoiding issues that may be of greater strategic importance.
7. Avoid becoming the dream interpreter.
   - This puts the power into the hands of the therapist.
8. Maintain an enquiring stance.
   - See the meaning of the dream as co-created.

9. Recall our own dreams, especially if prompted by a client the day before or the day after.
   - One study co-relates the therapist's active working on their own dreams in therapy with that of their clients (Schredl et al. 2000).
10. Dreams often occur at a point of transition in the client's psyche that is not visible or obvious in the current work.

Through on-going work with dreams, contemporary psychodynamic therapists have the opportunity to restore the place of dreams (and metaphors) as a vital aspect of our work. Working with clients' dreams is a privilege, like watching the carefree abandon and imagination of a child playing as we too get caught up in their world.

Bearing witness

Being alongside and bearing witness to another's psychic pain, and seeing release from this, is one of the most profound experiences of being a psychodynamic therapist. After Sherpa Tenzing and Edmund Hilary conquered Everest, on their descent the first person they met was another climber, George Lowe, who had climbed up to bring them some hot soup. Our clients conquer mountains in the internal range of the psyche. Sometimes our role is to be with them, at other times it is to offer hot soup and enable a safe descent after the exertion and exhaustion of a life-changing climb.

Climbers know that an accident is more likely to happen on the way down after a strenuous ascent. Clients invite us into their unformed traumas to help orientate them and to find a path through – or out of – the nightmare of an endless maze. For this they need a guide, but a guide who can bear witness to the depths of being human. The existential philosopher Martin Buber captures this well:

> The abyss does not call to his confidently functioning security of action, but to the abyss, that is to the self of the doctor, that selfhood that is hidden under the structures erected through training and practice, that is itself encompassed by chaos, itself familiar with demons, but is graced with the humble power of wrestling and overcoming, and is thus ready to wrestle and overcome ever anew.
>
> (Agassi 1999: 18–19)

Working dynamically, this is challenging, because many of the traumas we encounter in our clients are pre-verbal. (Perhaps we need to give clients a health warning that therapy can be traumatising.) Yet it is vital in order to accept the trauma or traumas (spoken and unspoken), and more importantly, the person experiencing it. Otherwise, the trauma becomes more important than the client and leaves them defined by events from the past.

Winnicott captures the idea of us failing our clients, but in their own way. They know, even if we fail them, we do so because we are human and because we have been with them with a non-defensive, blaming presence. A central therapeutic task therefore is to bear witness (Orange 2010). In a very real sense, therefore, suffering is an essential part of the therapeutic task. Davies (2011) argues that suffering is a vital part of our humanity and should not be seen as a problem to be medicalised or medicated, rather accepted as a fact of life that offers different ways of seeing and being in the world. This task of bearing witness and embracing suffering balances an apparently heroic form of martyrdom that could be masochist in nature, with an engagement in trauma that touches us but does not over-whelm us. Psychodynamic therapists, in being able to listen to the trauma of clients, even experiencing aspects of this themselves, give voice to silenced peoples and offer ways of holding together the shattered aspects of their lives. To enable us in this vital process, we need techniques that facilitate the life and growth of our clients and enable their aliveness to be encountered.

Attending to the spirit/soul

The psyche existed before Freud. In German, the word *seele*, coming from the Latin 'psy-che', can be translated as 'soul' or, after Freud, 'mind'. When Freud started at the University of Vienna, he was interested in philosophy (that included the soul) before taking up medi-cine. By the end of his time at university, the trajectory of Freud's thinking was empirical, evolutionary, scientific, non-religious, non-metaphysical, and non-mystical. Freud, in his passionate search for truth, wanted no distractions, no appeals to higher powers, no links to any agency external to the self, and no prohibitions upheld by religious traditions (1927).

In one sense, Freud was a flawed genius. We know more about the working of the mind, with his focus on unconscious processes, than had ever been dreamed. Freud, like many other thinkers, placed his faith in Modernity and the evolution of the human race through an absolute belief in rational thought. Yet at what cost? Historically, a dynamic approach to religious or spiritual experience was to view them as a failure of Oedipal development, an inappropriate dependence on a father (God), a symptom of psychopathology, and as a defence against standing on one's own two feet, though Pfister challenged this early on ([1928] 1993). This is changing, however (Ross 2006). Psychoanalysis and psychodynamic therapies have seen the emergence of spirituality as a vibrant part of their development in the last thirty years (Ross 2010). No longer do dynamic therapists, or their clients, need to put their soul outside the door of the consulting room. Importantly, spiritual phenomena can be found in the therapeutic process even when the therapist does not own a particular religious tradition (Ross 2016c, 2016d). Adopting a co-created intersubjective stance offers the idea that all of us, conscious and unconscious, spiritual and non-spiritual, are present and available for therapeutic engagement. The ideas of the transitional space and an ana-lytic third allow a new opportunity for engagement of the spirit or soul, influenced by vari-ous religious or spiritual traditions.

In order for a therapist to work with the whole client – body, mind, and soul – it is their responsibility to sign-post this at the assessment stage. Asking a question such as, 'Are there any spiritual or religious resources you draw on to help you manage?', reveals that this is an aspect that the client does not have to hide. Even more importantly, it enables the client to hear that they are being heard at their deepest level of being. The purpose of all therapy is for the client to grow and fulfil a potential they had not even realised was there.

Olivia's story

Olivia arrived for therapy looking terrified. She sat sobbing, shaking with emotion, looking like she might run for the door any second. Olivia was an actress but she reassured me she was not acting and this was no role she had ever sought. She came with a devoutly Christian faith but had begun to experience some disturbing flash-backs. Her minister referred her to me, as he believed I would be sympathetic to her background but not collusive with it. A history of terrible sexual abuse involving her father and mother emerged over two years of therapy.

Supervision was vital for me, as at times the negative transference to me as a minister of religion representing the God who had let her down was all-consuming. Olivia had tried therapy before but she felt her therapist believed her problems were compounded by her faith and the implicit message was she needed to give this up before she could make progress. Olivia left therapy and only came back because she believed I might be respectful to all of her – past and present, body, mind and soul. Olivia left therapy having made peace with her past (both parents had died and the trigger was sorting through the paperwork and the family home).

Ten years later, I received a letter telling me she had become a priest in the Church of England. She felt that the work done in therapy had been healing because it allowed her to be experienced as a broken but whole person. All our clients need that same opportunity, for us to attend to their soul.

Self-care

The need for self-care is not unique to therapists and has become an issue across all helping and teaching professions. Freud thought that we could never escape unscathed from wrestling with the demons of another's psyche. Jung coined the term 'wounded healer' to describe the therapeutic enterprise. Psychoanalytic developmental theorists expect a re-awakening and repeat of our earliest relationship, for good or ill, in our demanding therapeutic work (Beebe and Lachmann 2014). Bollas imagines that to discover the psyche of the client, we need to search in our own psyche (1987), itself a daunting and relentless task.

Dealing with these demands is an essential task in our work. As therapists, we have an ethical responsibility for the well-being of our clients, which we can fulfil by looking after *our* well-being. As dynamic therapists, subject to multiple transferential and projective processes, there is an even greater need to attend to our self-care and develop the emotional resilience required by this kind of work. Being on the receiving end of projections, client after client, day after day, can be wearying. All therapists, of whatever background, can find it difficult when they are working with clients whose life stories and traumas touch on their own. At one level, it gives additional insight; at another, it adds further complications. Supervision plays a crucial role in helping therapists attend to their self-care and work through any such complication (Wheeler 2007).

We can begin with a number of simple steps, including:

- a healthful diet;
- the right amount of sleep;
- periods of relaxation, including planned breaks and holidays;
- physical exercise;
- mental exercise;

- reading;
- journalling;
- maintaining friendships; and
- meditative practices, including mindfulness and prayer.

There are some advanced steps that also make a great deal of difference.

- The first is learning to say 'no', not just to the things we don't want to do – that's easy – but to the things we want to do.
  - One of my colleagues commented that they felt I gave my time away too easily. They were not complaining, because they and the students benefitted, but they wondered at what cost to me.
- The second is living in the rhythm of life as it is, not as it once was.
  - In my mountain climbing activities with my son, I have to remember I am not his age. I cannot do what I once did. My climbing accident has left my ankles less flexible and my knees more arthritic. So too, as a therapist, I cannot do the hours I once did or switch from task to task, or client to client. I now take time to transition in and out. I therefore leave longer spaces between clients so I can hold them in mind, before and after each session, allowing me to take care both of them and myself.

Short-term working

What difference does time make? Where do time-limited psychodynamic therapies fit in this broader context of change (Coren 2010, 2016; Hobson 2016)?

Freud (1937) recognised psychoanalysis was time-consuming and saw the danger it could become interminable. In the histories of psychoanalysis, psychotherapy, and counselling (Chapter 2), battle-lines were drawn around the length, frequency, and implied depth of each approach. The dilemma is that many therapists working in the NHS or voluntary contexts have to work with time-limited models. When working in a university context, I am constantly amazed how much progress student clients can make in relatively few sessions because of their particular stage of growth and development. When working in private practice, I am all too aware that clients need much more therapy than they can afford. In any context, dynamic therapists continue to think psychodynamically, even if we do not have the opportunity to do more than connect the past with the present, and the mind with the body, emotions, and soul.

The analytic tradition set a precedent for working long-term with clients, although that is not the whole story; Freud did see brief cases and one-off consultations (Ross 2016e). Since the development of focal, brief, or time-limited dynamic therapies, initiated by Balint, Malan (1979), and many other early colleagues, psychodynamic principles and practice have been applied in fewer and fewer sessions. These range from four to sixteen sessions, though six has become the default number in our cost-conscious times (Coren 2010). Currently, the main contenders are:

- Psychodynamic Interpersonal Therapy (PIT, also called the Conversational Model) (Barkham et al. 2016);
- Cognitive Analytic Therapy (CAT);

- Interpersonal Therapy (IPT);
- Intensive Short-Term Dynamic Psychotherapy (ISTDP);
- Dynamic Interpersonal Therapy (DIT) (Lemma et al. 2011); and
- Brief Psychoanalytic Therapy (BPT) (Hobson 2016).

All have their strengths and all use research evidence to demonstrate their effectiveness. Short-term working requires a number of changes to the way therapists engage with their longer-term, open-ended clients.

- First, you work with the end in mind from the very beginning. No one likes endings but it provides the opportunity to focus.
- Second, at assessment, decisions need to made as to what the key focus of the work is going to be. This is no archaeological dig of the psyche looking for buried remains from the past, rather a quick skim over the surface with a metal detector. Both can find treasure.
- Third, there is often less opportunity to work with transference, counter-transference, projections, or co-created intersubjectivities. These take time and trust to emerge.
- Fourth, the therapist needs to be more pro-active in establishing the working alliance, and more directive in the therapy itself.
- Fifth, the therapist needs to assess whether the nature of the client's difficulties admit of being addressed ethically within the time-frame available. A client working through bereavement may well find six sessions very helpful. Another client with a history of abuse (of whatever kind) may find six sessions unhelpful as this will barely scratch the surface.
- Sixth, it may require a more experienced therapist to work short-term. Trainees (who receive less than weekly supervision) may have only just got hold of the client before they are gone.

The key aim is to do simple psychodynamic things well: connecting the past with the present; bringing to attention what is not being said; voicing feelings in the room; and enabling the client to tell their story and find their voice. Short-term work is more demanding than longer-term work, with the pressure on the therapist to get things right the very first time. In longer-term work, if you miss something, the client has the time to remind you. If there is an impasse or rupture, there is time to try and resolve this.

Summary

The skill of assessment grows as we become more experienced, and this offers the opportunity do more and more through this aspect of the therapeutic process. This includes recognising and working with projective and intersubjective processes; working with dreams and metaphors; attending to the soul; before bearing witness and finally ending the relationship. Two further subjects we explored included the need for self-care and the demands brought about by working short-term. These form part of the skills we require to be dynamic therapists.

The next chapter will examine how our use of psychodynamic therapy, how our application of these skills, changes people.

Reflective questions

What are you going to do in the next week to improve your self-care?

How do you need to adjust your therapeutic stance in working with short-term clients? Are you trying to do too much?

Looking at research

Douglas Thomas, *Dreams and Evidence-based Practice: The empirical case for restoring dream work to best therapeutic practices.* Available at:

http://drdouglasthomas.com/DT_images/WRITING_Dreams&EBP.pdf [accessed 31 July 2018].

15

Therapeutic engagement and the process of change

Having reached the base camp of contemporary psychodynamic therapy, we can look back and scan the horizon below to see where we have come from. The variegated landscape reveals the many paths and crossing points we have traversed. We can look up as the summit ahead beckons, calling us on for the final push. There is excitement that we are further in our therapeutic sojourn than we have ever been before. What drives us forward is a passion to know others at depth, bringing help and hope. While these are not always possible in practice, it is what motivates us. The complicated part is that we, and the client, need to be prepared to change. Clients come to therapy *thinking* they want to change but discover it is difficult. Even when thoughts, feelings, and memories disturb us, we resist. We rationalise, we fear risk, we avoid loss, and we settle for the known rather than face the unknown. Change is often dislocating and disturbing yet is a normal part of life. Contemporary psychodynamic therapy, encompassing new ideas, research, and clinical practices, encourages change.

This chapter focuses on what shape psychodynamic engagement takes and how this facilitates change. In one sense, this chapter can never be complete because we begin and end therapy with clients we rarely or never see or hear from again. What we can say is that, by the end of therapy, the emotional trajectory of most clients is upwards as they are launched into a new phase of life. Honesty requires me to say that some clients do not substantially improve despite their, and my, best efforts. Here we learn together about accepting limitations and mourning loss.

So how does psychodynamic therapy change people?

Engaging with the unconscious

Contemporary psychodynamic therapy, like classical psychoanalysis, has the unconscious at the heart of all it does. If you buy a ring made of precious metal, on the inside of the band there are hallmarks showing the manufacturer; the quality of the gold, silver, or platinum; where it was assayed (authorised); and the year it was made. Contemporary psychodynamic therapy only needs one hallmark, the unconscious, as the stamp of authenticity and authority. Many other therapies borrow techniques from psychodynamic therapy but it is only here that we can fully experience the depth of unconscious processes.

In Chapter 5, we saw how Freud believed the purpose of psychoanalysis was to make the unconscious conscious, and to establish the ego (rather than the id or the super-ego) as the central agent in the psyche. For many clients, understanding what is happening and giving them choice are crucial ways of gaining control over aspects of life that are troubling.

Janet (who we saw in Chapter 13) was looking for insight into her unconscious patterns and motivations. While such insights do not guarantee repeating old patterns, they minimise their automatic repetition. Clients come to dynamic therapy because they want to discover and work with the unconscious.

Being the right person at the right time

With some clients, all I do is set light to the touch-paper and they rocket off, exploding (in a good way) in vibrant colour across the dark sky. With others, the matches are damp, the touch-paper fizzles at first but then expires. The rocket remains inert, silently accusing, with disappointed spectators still waiting and hoping. Another attempt (against safety advice) and *whoosh*, the disappointment turns to delight. Some clients are ready to engage with a psychodynamic way of working that fits where they are and encounter a therapist that seems to fit with them. Some clients build an immediate working alliance that is strong enough to bear the pressures of defences, resistances, transferences, mistakes, and breaks in the therapeutic frame. Either way, this cannot be manufactured or pre-programmed and reminds us therapy involves two unique people, and two unique unconsciousnesses. This explains why people seek therapy and are willing to pay – they value the choice of finding someone with whom they feel at home. In publicly funded contexts, you get who you get and this is 'good-enough', which can limit the effectiveness of the therapeutic encounter but underlines the importance of the assessment stage to ensure there is a right fit between client and therapist.

Discovering emotional insight and personal agency

Many clients (and some therapists) are disconnected from their emotions. Emotions are a foreign language we seek to master, having realised the limitations of our emotional phrasebook. When asking the waiter for a dessert, using my best Italian by uttering the phrase 'crème calamari', I had him laughing and crying. Thankfully, I shut up and pointed to the menu instead. Clients come to therapy being able to point at emotions where they are, as yet, just words on a page. They are not deeply felt parts of their experience (with complex causes originating in their family of origin). Therapy enables clients to find an emotional vocabulary, put this into words, and voice a narrative that frees them.

Paula's story

In session five (of six), Paula stammered, 'I didn't know I felt like that'. Decades of sadness poured out in a deluge of pain and loss. It was a profound moment of emotional insight that made sense of long-buried feelings. Given our limited number of sessions, there is more work Paula can do in the future (around anger) but in the moment this was enough. She had discovered an emotional connection in herself and new words and feelings to express them.

It was just such emotional connections Freud made with his earliest clients that launched psychoanalysis (1893–1895). Such connections develop personal agency and the ability to tell one's narrative with a sense of personal participation (Pollock and Slavin 1998). Personal agency moves us from being the actor waiting in the wings onto the centre of the stage. Personal agency is to see the bright lights and perform for the audience but crucially requires the experience of one's self as an agent in one's own life and perceptions. This requires sufficient parental and developmental processes and it explains why early trauma and abuse are so destructive. It requires a person to be a person with a self that acts in the service of them, not others. The clients who struggle with personal agency are the ones whose trauma is hidden. On the surface, they appear fine, but digging deeper you often discover they have grown up with a narcissistic mother. Digging deeper requires us to be ever alert to clues, hints, and disconnections, aware that whatever is happening on the surface is not all that it seems. In terms of transference, there is the repetition from early childhood that the client feels they have to meet our need by being a 'good' client. The early messages they received were that they exist as an object that reflects the mother and meets her needs, rather than the mother enabling the baby to become their own person.

Discovering new narratives and unlocking metaphors

When clients discover a new emotional vocabulary, this is used to revisit their life-story. The work of transference, in all its forms, allows the client to re-author aspects of their life. For some, it is a discovery of how emotionally deprived their past was. We take our own experience as the norm even if we know it was distorted or damaging. Survival meant that some thoughts or feelings were stored away like an unwanted Christmas present, too precious to pass on to a charity shop, but of no value in the moment. They lurk in darkness and dust, waiting to be unwrapped.

When I was 40, I avoided a mid-life crisis (although I did change career), but I felt impelled to write about my past (Ross 1997). Therapy illuminated my narrative, made new emotional connections and unleashed the unconscious. It released unspoken ties that had bound me, allowing me to make sense of myself. I also completed a psychodynamic therapy training programme (with Michael Jacobs and Moira Walker), which was reparative and illuminating. By examining my old narratives, I was able to create new narratives (in the form of a book), allowing them to be accessible to others. Twenty years later, I still get letters and emails and meet people who tell me that my story has reflected their story and been of great help at key moments in their life. Yet it has had its costs, which I could not have known at the time.

What also happens in therapy is a discovery of new metaphors that unlock something unexpected in us. Part of the therapeutic task is to find the right metaphor for the client, which requires attunement on our part. Sometimes, clients suggest something that comes from a dream but resonates and grows throughout the therapy. Emmanuel Levinas saw the value of metaphor lying in the capacity to take us beyond the literal meaning, like an invitation to the transcendent, evoking a whole new order of meaning. Like Lacan (1977: 247f.), I believe metaphors open up new dimensions of meaning that are hidden. Winnicott took the child's game of hide and seek very seriously, telling us that in our hiddenness, it is a disaster never to be found (Winnicott 1965; Ogden 2001).

Metaphors remind us we exist in a paradox of presence, absence, hiddenness, and discovery, each metaphor giving us the opportunity to discover a new meaning, to meet a new absence and encounter another aspect of our hiddenness. Dynamic therapy enables us to use metaphors in a uniquely novel way, where they become a tool for exploring less-visited parts of the psyche. The psyche itself is a metaphor for all that goes on in the mind that we cannot comprehend or measure, existing out of awareness. Winnicott used the metaphor of a psychiatric hospital to explain an aspect of the true self.

> . . . the true self is hidden right away and only emerges under very special conditions if at all . . . the patient turns himself into a mental hospital and the true self is a patient hidden away in the back somewhere in a padded cell.
>
> (quoted in Rodman 1987: 81)

This metaphor tells me so much more about the true self and how, as a therapist, I need to help clients find this aspect of themselves. I need to be careful and slow, negotiating locked wards, facing disturbing figures (in our past and present), with a special kind of holding and containment.

Holding and containment

When I first encountered these ideas as clinical practices, they made sense at some deep unspoken level. As Slochower wisely says, 'Holding creates room. It establishes space in which experience of the self and other deepen' (2014: 1). It was as if this metaphor opened a space in my mind and my psyche for another person. Clients can legitimately ask, 'What is it that is being held?', 'How am I being contained?', 'Why do I need these things?'. Holding and being held are elemental to life.

The brain scans of babies who have rarely or never been touched, held, or cuddled show gaps in their brains like neural black holes. Winnicott takes holding as a living metaphor from our earliest good-enough mother–baby interactions that shape the emergent psyche and the development of the brain (see Chapter 10).

When I was trapped on a rocky ledge after my fall, it was so affirming to be held by the paramedic dropped from a helicopter to rescue me. His firm but gentle touch to determine what parts of me weren't broken was life-affirming (Ross 2014, 2016a).

We create a holding space in psychodynamic therapy through the rhythm of meeting in the same place and the same time (wherever possible), and with the same welcome for the client in our mind or psyche, facing whatever they bring. Many of our clients, and a fair few therapists, have not had good-enough holding. Holding is less physical and more *psychical*, as if the unconscious of the other, the client, knows they are in the presence of someone who wants to address all aspects of their being. This includes the furtive, shameful, damaged, broken, betrayed, and unspeakable experience of the abyss that many encounter but never talk about. It is as if we are helicoptered in to reach the remote part of their psyche where they feel trapped and unable to move, which if left, becomes a psychic form of death.

Together these combine to form what has been called a 'holding environment' (Finlay 2016; Lemma 2016) or a form of analytic holding (Casement 1985). The phrase that is often associated is 'holding in mind'.

Just as a mother does not forget her baby, remembering to feed, change, or soothe them, therapists do not forget their clients. This happens at two levels. The first is being ready for the client's session, which if forgotten indicates that some other unconscious dynamic is at work that needs to be addressed. The second is a wondering about where a client might be now and how they are getting on. I still miss my Monday five o'clock client (see Izzy, Chapter 14). Partly, because it was a time-slot I have only ever used for that client. Another part is because when she left, our work was unfinished and her need for rehab was a greater priority. Holding and containment can be the precursors required to enable clients to move towards the mutuality found in the best intersubjective encounters and gives personal agency for continuing being.

Mentalisation and affect regulation

Mentalising is a skill we learn as infants when all has gone well. As we are attended to, nourished, and cared for, we develop a secure sense of self with secure attachments. As *we* have been attuned to, we are enabled to attune to others. My work with Kat (Chapter 7) involved getting her to hold in mind what other people might be thinking or feeling about what she might say or do. It was as if some words in her emotional vocabulary were missing. Yet with practice, using therapy as a learning space, she was able to do this attuning with increasing accuracy. This had a beneficial impact in terms of her impulse control and suicidal actions, sadly without these being removed altogether. Bateman and Fonagy (2004, 2016) pioneered mentalisation, underpinned by research for effectiveness with particular client groups (2008); however, the principles also apply to other areas of mental health (2011).

Mentalising is also helpful in getting clients to work with their thinking and feelings connected to trauma. Most clients are able to mentalise to a degree but therapy offers an opportunity for this to be enhanced. This helps clients understand their affects as a range of powerful feelings. Knowing how these operate gives the option of control over their expression (Fonagy et al. 2004). A growing emotional vocabulary allows a greater knowledge as to what is appropriate and in what context.

Malc's story

Malc was a very angry man who threatened to hit his partner, Adam, when they became locked into an argument that seemed to spiral out of control. Therapy enabled Malc to connect with the powerlessness of his own childhood and feelings of abandonment (his mother left him in the care of an alcoholic and violent father).

Malc realised how he was repeating an abusive pattern he had experienced. He had nobody reliable to teach him how to mentalise, to think and feel what the other person might be thinking or feeling, when he lashed out verbally. Adam was not a source of comfort, or so Malc thought, until he began to see the fear in Adam, who withdrew in order to protect himself. Malc realised that he was causing this, so rather than getting angry, he began to talk about his newly discovered emotions that threatened to overwhelm him.

Malc found individual therapy helpful and this enabled him to face the prospect of couples' counselling to attend to other issues.

Moments of meeting

We all know a moment of meeting when we experience it with our clients or in our own therapy. Various unique connections happen where we feel as if something deep has been touched in us, even at the depths of our soul, that some understand as activating an archetypal or transpersonal encounter (Kalsched 2013). Drawing on Stern and the BCPSG (2010), we now know this is a repeat and a repair drawn from our earliest experiences. These may be expressed in terms of spiritual phenomena (Ross 2016c, 2016d), but they echo the most profound mother–baby encounters. These moments of meeting serve as springboards, enabling us to dive deeper into our own psyche and the psyche of another, forming the first step in an intersubjective process.

Steph's story

Steph ('Don't call me Stephanie, I think you are telling me off') was finding her young daughter, Ruby, was stirring long-forgotten feelings. I made a comment similar to 'When you tell me about Ruby, I think you are telling me about yourself when you were Ruby's age', adding intuitively, 'but you can't tell anyone as you fear nobody will believe you'. The effect of this comment was alarming, as if Steph had been given an electric shock. She sat bolt upright in the chair and stared at me, mesmerised, asking 'How did you know?'

Steph realised I didn't think she was mad and instead believed what she was saying, so she told me more, bringing disturbing dreams to each session. I would listen and make connections about what she was saying, but more importantly about what was *not* being said, capturing the texture of the dream. In one dream, she was trapped inside a building crashing to the ground following an earthquake. In another, she saw herself playing on a roundabout going faster and faster until it spun off into the sky, depositing her alone on a barren moonscape. She could breathe but nobody else was there. Utterly alone, she wept desolately but nobody came to rescue her. Steph offered her own interpretation:

'When I was four (the age of her daughter now), we had a new neighbour who was very friendly. He offered to babysit and one night he touched me where he shouldn't and made me touch him. He told me it was our secret. I was scared, excited, and confused. If I told anyone he said nobody would believe me. I kept that secret until he moved away years later. I told my mum but she shouted at me for saying such horrible things about our kind ex-neighbour'.

What released her forgotten past was a moment of meeting where Steph felt heard at a deep, unspoken level.

Rupture and repair

Just as every successful therapy has moments of meeting, it also has moments of rupture. Things can and do go wrong. We call the client the wrong name (remember Wendy from Chapter 3?); we forget an important event; we mistime an interpretation, which makes the client feel they have not been heard; we fail to connect some vital aspect of the past. The ways in which we as therapists can hinder the therapeutic process could stretch on and on, which only goes to illustrate our frailty and humanity.

Over 75 years ago, Ferenczi suggested that admitting our mistakes creates confidence in the therapeutic relationship and validates the experience of the client (Pollock and Slavin 1998: 865). In Chapter 13, we saw how spotting ruptures and taking the actions required to repair these were crucial in clients completing therapy. The experience of both is vital.

In one of my early experiences of therapy, I plucked up enough courage to say that I did not feel I was being heard. The therapist agreed he had been pre-occupied (without elaborating about what) and indicated that he would now attend to me properly. This gave me the affirmation that my own thoughts and feelings were valid. We continued for some time after this in what I felt was a helpful experience. On another occasion, a different supervisor seemed to ignore what I said, which I repeated only to be told that the purpose of supervision was to focus on clinical work, not personal issues. I had raised it because, for me as a supervisor, I attend to the whole person, which includes what is going on in their real, *personal* world. While this supervision had been very helpful in the past, it will come as no surprise that we parted ways shortly afterwards occasioned by my changing circumstances. Both were ruptures, but only one was repaired.

Attending to splits and integrating disowned aspects

Splitting is a powerful psychic defence that we all use, consciously and unconsciously, in individuals, couples, families, groups, and institutions. Originating in Klein, it is a term used more widely and, in an extreme form, appears psychotic. Bion explained this as the impact of bizarre, disintegrated objects that inhabit the psyche (Grotstein 2007). At its simplest level, we all have things about ourselves we like and don't like. In a powerful training exercise, I asked students to identify which part of their body they liked and which part they did not like. This revealed, in an embodied way, how we split into good versus bad all the time but rarely think about it.

Jasmin's story

Jasmin was a 23-year-old fitness instructor when she developed cancer. As a consequence of chemotherapy, her hair fell out. She came to me depressed. 'Look at me' she said, pointing to her short pixie-style hair. 'This is not me. All my curls have gone'.

Jasmin explained that she had always had a large curly head of hair, which formed a part of herself she loved. Now it was gone. The therapy was not about celebrating living and overcoming illness, rather mourning and loss, the loss of the 'self' Jasmin felt she had been.

Several years later, I unexpectedly met Jasmin in a social context. When I end with clients, we agree that if we ever meet, it is up to them if they wish to approach me. I will not ignore them on purpose but try to respect their space and who they might be with. In a quiet moment, Jasmin came up to me and said quietly so no one else would hear, 'I like my hair now', smiled and walked away. It was a curiously intimate moment but it was all I needed to know; she was well in her outer and inner worlds.

It can be a struggle to own the aspects of us that are challenging such as ruthlessness, aggression, darkness, and despair. Therapy enables disowned aspects of the self and our defensive splits to be identified and come to terms with, even if never fully accepted. It also touches on releasing embodied trauma. My experience of embodied trauma following a life-threatening fall was about a depth of engagement at an archetypal and unconscious level. My body, mind, psyche, and soul needed attention to recover and enable me to regain the health and well-being I possess today. D.H. Lawrence, whose writing is rich with embodiment, viewed our flesh and blood as wiser than our mind. He believed it was in the unconscious forms of embodiment that we discover the depths of our soul and, beyond that, the wider cosmos (1921).

Difference, diversity, and otherness

Martin Luther King, Jr. was a unique combination of visionary, dreamer, and activist. His words still echo with a power and resonance that captures our attention.

> [We are] caught in an inescapable network of mutuality. And whatever affects one directly affects all indirectly. For some strange reason, I can never be what I ought to be until you are what you ought to be. And you can never be what you ought to be until I am what I ought to be. This is the way God's universe is made; this is the way it is structured.

> (1968)

Sharing King's vision and influenced by relational psychoanalysis and intersubjective perspectives, contemporary psychodynamic therapy sees working with difference, diversity, and otherness as an essential part of the therapeutic task (Wheeler 2006).

In simple terms, the fault-line that separates classical understandings of psychoanalysis and psychodynamic therapies from contemporary understandings is that of dealing with difference and diversity. The real world where people live out who they are confronts us, often uncomfortably so, with issues of power, inclusion, exclusion, marginalisation, and victimisation, leading to rejection and discrimination. If these issues are not addressed, we rob people of their essential humanity. Addressing such issues forms a core part of the values enshrined in the BACP's *Ethical Framework for the Counselling Professions* (2018).

My otherness in relation to psychoanalytic and psychodynamic thinking is that I am part of a Christian faith tradition, engage in spiritual practices, and see the soul as an essential part of the psyche. Historically, such beliefs have been viewed as pathological, a failure to fully resolve an Oedipal complex, and sufficient to prevent me from training as a psychoanalyst. Yet my experiences are infinitesimally small compared with the prejudice so many of my colleagues and clients have experienced because of their race, gender, disability, and sexual orientation. Martin Luther King, Jr.'s dream still needs to be dreamed in a slow march of progress in order to counter-balance the nightmare scenarios that present themselves with narratives of threat or suspicion. It is no longer sufficient to be part of a status quo resting on laurels from the past. Contemporary psychodynamic therapy locates itself on the cutting-edge of new forms of engagement with life-enhancing forms of difference, diversity, and otherness.

Shaking things loose

The effect of therapy is to shake us up – in a good way. We can only say that after the event, as in the moment it feels overwhelming and we want it to stop. What gets shaken are our conscious and unconscious processes, our well-honed rationalisations and defences, our complacencies and unspoken collusions, and our motivations. The 'facts' about ourselves we thought we knew are laid bare, stripped of disguise or subterfuge. In becoming vulnerable, we need a therapist that makes it safe by holding the therapeutic frame, possessing ethical mindedness, and maintaining professional standards and a commitment to our well-being. Sometimes things come loose easily, as if we know it is time to let such memories, or traumas, go. Other times things need a great deal of effort to prise open. Just like barnacles attached to a hull, these need to be removed from the mind, body, psyche, and soul to reveal what is underneath and restore us to our fullest state of functioning. Dynamic therapy is not an easy process but it offers a place and a relationship where the unsayable can be said, the unthinkable thought, through the agency of another. Freud shook the foundations of our thinking about the mind in the nineteenth and twentieth centuries; contemporary psychodynamic therapy shakes the foundations for the twenty-first century and beyond.

Faith, hope, love, and tenderness

St. Paul concludes one of the best-known New Testament passages (1 Corinthians 13) with a sustained meditation on love, focusing on the profoundest meeting conceivable, 'face to face', between a created person and their Creator, adding 'there remains faith, hope and love, these three, and the greatest of these *is* love' (my translation and emphasis). The love implied here comes from the Greek *agape*, meaning an extravagant delight in the other, rather than *eros*, which is much more focused on the self and from which we get the term 'erotic' (see C.S. Lewis's classic text *The Four Loves* [1960]). Meng believed it was this expression of love that united Freud in his unlikely friendship with a Swiss Protestant Pastor, Oskar Pfister, with whom he maintained a lifelong correspondence from their first meeting in 1909.

> At the root of both lay love of the truth, indeed love itself, as the central factor in obtaining an understanding of mankind.
>
> (1963: 9)

In what ways does contemporary psychodynamic therapy offer faith, hope, and love? To this tripartite way of being I believe we should add tenderness. How do these all-too-often ignored aspects change our clients?

Faith

A feature of a many clients' experience is that they have lost a belief in themselves. The fact that they are with someone who believes them, and believes they can find a way through, is another example of personal agency and this forges something of immense value in the molten core of their being. It is analogous to that most basic trust between mother and baby that Winnicott writes so eloquently about. While Bion talked about 'acts of faith', and Winnicott spoke of 'areas of faith', I want to add into this heady mix a new idea based on the 'phenomenology of faith'. Psychodynamic therapy ceases to be dynamic unless faith is present, faith in the theories elaborated over decades and generations, in the clinical practices that have evolved as we learn from clients and see beyond the confines of culture, in the person who is the client in all their pain and potentiality, and finally in the possibility of something new being created in and through this encounter. This involves the following stages.

1. *The phenomenology of the unconscious.* It requires an act of faith to evoke the unconscious because like all unconscious processes, they are unconscious and may or may not present in some way. I wonder if over time we come to sense the unconscious, feeling it in our bodies, sensing it in neural pathways, or experience a ripple of movement at a subliminal level, a stirring of the soul and whether it is these faith-filled experiences that spark intuition. The paradox is, the greater the depth of thinking and reflecting, the more intuitive we become.

2. *The phenomenology of dreaming.* As explored in the previous chapter, we can now develop a broader understanding of what happens in and through dreaming. Dreams are less disguised than Freud originally suggested. We need to live the dream as an expression of our being. This is a step that requires faith, conviction to stay in the now, and not to try to find some secret knowledge the dream reveals. Instead, we can focus on a recovery of the idea of dreams as revelatory. But the revelation is about ourselves experienced in a new way. This allows dreams to open out back in time, and go beyond time. They offer a connection to oneself, to one's spirit or soul often in connection to the other.

3. *The phenomenology of intersubjective creativity.* Something happens in therapy. What we call it varies and is found across all therapeutic modalities. It is variously termed: 'magic', 'mystical', 'wholeness', 'unity', 'transpersonal', 'transcendent', 'otherness', 'love', 'moment of meeting', 'relational depth', or 'immanent or transcendent empathy'. Martin Buber's (1958) concept of the I-Thou put words to the phenomena in terms of a form of

connectedness at a depth that encompasses the soul. Buber calls us to have faith that moves us from a static I-It place into the dynamic I-Thou experience.

4. *The phenomenology of spirit/soul and the other*. What happens when therapy takes us somewhere else? The encounters we experience in therapy can be agonising.

Milly's story

A former client, Milly, told me about her being groomed when she was just 15. I was the first person she told.

She wanted to be rid of this so her 'spirit can be free'. Notice the soul-laden language. But setting her spirit free is slow and painful work. It takes faith on her part to enter into a process she cannot know the outcome of. It feels like a painstaking restoration of an old but treasured car, where the psychic rust can be stripped away and restored to its former glory. More organically, it is like the growing of a plant from seed, sheltered through the winter in a greenhouse, waiting for the day to be planted and to grow in a garden, thus revealing the beauty of shape and flower in due season. These are the evolutions of faith that are part of our contemporary psychodynamic work. They also touch on hope.

Hope

Hope is a late arrival to the psychoanalytic party although an important idea in contemporary psychodynamic thinking (Casement 1990). It clusters around two central ideas. The first is that one of the roles of the therapist is to hold onto hope, whatever the client brings. Even if in despair and the client has no hope to offer for themselves, they sense that their therapist holds onto a hope, no matter how fragmentary, that things can be different. This is not a passive form of wishful thinking (as that wouldn't do justice to the client's trauma), rather it is an active stance by the therapist. The second is that hope comes by acknowledging the pain, loss, tragedy, suffering, and psychopathology as in this act there is a discovery that hope can still be present. In the words of one of Winnicott's patients, who he helped to move from their false self to their true self,

> The only time I felt hope was when you told me you could see no hope, and you continued with the analysis.

> (1965: 152)

Similarly, Mitchell, in writing about hope and dread in analysis, emphasised that we need both to be present to overcome the over-emphasis on hope in self-psychology and the over-emphasis of dread in Kleinian thinking. In bringing them together, a new form of thinking emerges, we enter into a dancing landscape and experience the dialectics of hope (Mitchell 1993). One of the outcomes of being held or contained is that within oneself there is a capacity to hope, whatever external circumstances bring. It is like an expression of love.

Love and tenderness

Barsness (2018) and colleagues identify eight core competencies in relational psychoanalysis. These overlap with the ideas developed in this book that form the heart of contemporary psychodynamic therapy, yet there was one core competency that hit home just like Eros's arrow: the word 'Love'. This is a rarely talked about subject in psychoanalysis that speaks to the heart of being human. Freud wrote about the psychology of love (spanning 1910–1918) but added little insight or wisdom other than the importance of transference-love (see Chapter 13). Controversially, Sayers argues that the losses experienced by Freud, especially of those he loved, led to his rejection of deep human connection, 'dismissing as an illusion the oneness with another of being in love, and the oceanic oneness with the otherness of God or the universe of religious and mystical experience' (2003: 60).

Bion offers greater insight when he talks about the complexities of love and refers to an absolute love that transcends language (López-Corvo 2003: 166), something we all feel at an intuitive level. Love in the twenty-first century is variously romanticised, trivialised, agonised, sexualised, fantasised, traumatised, or simply absent. It is what people want irrespective of whether they become clients and it sets the context of all therapeutic work. Freud was both romantic, writing thousands of passionate love-letters to Martha his fiancé, and pragmatic, believing we live to work and love. So loving others in a way that does not possess, control, manipulate, or eroticise, and in a way that offers trust, faith, hope, belief, intimacy, and belonging forms the granite-like foundations we all need.

In the previous chapter, we examined the power and importance of transference-love and the problems that arise when this is eroticised, yet this should not divert us from the task of loving ourselves, and our clients, with a passion. We can help clients to love again, receiving and giving to others in the place of absence or abuse. We can help clients disentangle the knots of confusion about what it is to love and to take risks in expressing the depth of our being. We can help clients recover bonds of love that bind others and us together in a unique way enabling us to be human, individually and collectively.

A unique way in which that love can be expressed by psychodynamic therapists is through the capacity for, and expression of, tenderness. For the last five years, I have met with a group of British psychoanalysts at the New Imago conference held in Oxford annually. Interdisciplinary in nature, it is a group of people committed to a psychoanalytic way of thinking, but what strikes me most is how thoughtful, compassionate, and tender they are when talking about their work and their patients. This is so far removed from the much-caricatured 'blank screen' of classical psychoanalysis. While tenderness remains a taboo subject, McCulloch (2009) draws together analytic and philosophical thinking from Ferenczi, Suttie, Balint, and Barthes to argue for a recovery of tenderness. Such tenderness requires authenticity, which is enhanced when engaging in a co-created intersubjective meeting. Like McCulloch, I believe that an important goal of psychodynamic therapeutic processes is to enable the client to discover both their toughness and their tenderness, and the therapist models this to them. This offers the client the possibility of avoiding splits and fostering integration.

While my broken body was on a trolley in a hospital emergency trauma ward, being examined for a head injury and multiple breaks and fractures, a nurse asked if there was anything she could do. I said that my toes were cold (having had the beginning stages of hypothermia). Gently she massaged my toes, bringing them warmth. This touch was so tender it did something powerful to me, as if catapulted back in time to being a helpless baby needing the comforting touch of another when in distress.

What we do in psychodynamic therapy can range from life-saving surgery to massaging frozen toes, restoring circulation to a broken body, psyche, and soul. Often we do both in bringing people alive and re-connecting them with their aliveness of being. For some clients, this begins with us seeing it within them and offering ways in which it can be encountered.

A last word

Over my life, I have discovered that I am attracted to empty spaces that have stood the test of time with a patina of age, an untold history of human connection – wild landscapes, mountains, Neolithic stones, dolmen and circles, early medieval churches, derelict asylum hospitals, abstract art and, paradoxically, dreams. Such places, structures, and artefacts possess an innate structure and fecundity of being that inflames the imagination. They generate experiences of paradox – aloneness and connection, safety and risk, elemental and spiritual. It is these qualities that are incarnated in the best psychodynamic and integrative therapists, supervisors, trainers, and researchers. My hope is that you will come to believe you belong here too.

In this book, we have moved from chaos, through complexity, into a dancing landscape characterised by creativity and connections. In writing about contemporary psychodynamic counselling and psychotherapy, I have chosen to be conversational and personal. It reflects who I am and offers you the space to create your own version that best reflects your unique being, whilst also being grounded in the wisdom of the past.

Key thinkers

Wilfred Bion (1897–1974)

Bion served with distinction as an officer in a Tank Battalion during the First World War, but the experience was traumatic. He went on to study history and literature and acquired interests in philosophy and art. Training as a doctor, Bion specialised in psychiatry and focused on psychoanalysis with a post at the Tavistock Clinic. During the Second World War, as a Major in the army, he worked alongside Rickman (his analyst) in developing innovative group work at Northfield Military Hospital, Birmingham, which was continued after the War at the Tavistock (see *Experience in Groups* [1961]). He went into analysis with Klein and developed pioneering ideas in working with psychotic or borderline patients including alpha and beta elements, the Grid, containment, transformations in O, faith, K, nameless dread, and many others. He built on Freud and incorporated Klein's ideas in his unique synthesis. Later in his career, he went to Los Angeles where he influenced a new generation of psychoanalysts including Grotstein (2007) and his writing became more personal and more edgy. His seminars in South America were also very influential and enabled the spread of psychoanalysis beyond its Western European origins.

John Bowlby (1907–1990)

Bowlby came from an upper-middle-class English family that upheld the social conventions of the day about bringing up children. From birth onwards, a nanny would be employed to do the day-to-day tasks, and as the child grew they would be allowed an hour or so with the mother, often between tea and bedtime. Bowlby thought that the loss of a caring, loving nanny for a child up to the age of five was a tragedy equal to the death of a mother. At the age of eight, children were sent away to boarding school, returning only for occasional weekends and school holidays. Bowlby endured this but felt profoundly unhappy, like entering into a dark tunnel, where each term felt like an endless trauma of separation from home and the relationships this represents. Bowlby believed that while he had been hurt by these experiences, he had not been irreparably damaged. We can clearly see here the origins of his later thinking on attachment, separation, and loss. Training as a doctor and a psychoanalyst, Bowlby was influenced as a scientist by Lorenz and focused on the early attachment patterns that could be seen in mothers and babies. Other colleagues, including

Ainsworth, and Main enabled the development of attachment theory, which has provided a rich vein of research (Fonagy 2001).

Erik Erikson (1902–1994)

Erikson's mother was Danish, his father unknown, so to avoid a scandal she moved to Germany before he was born. Brought up Jewish by his mother and step-father, Erikson later converted to Christianity. A friend, Peter Blos, invited him to Vienna to help teach in a private school set up by Dorothy Burlingham (heiress to the Tiffany fortune) and work with Anna Freud. Here, Erikson trained as a child analyst, and was in personal analysis with Anna. He emigrated first to Denmark, then to Boston, USA in 1933, becoming the first child psychoanalyst. Erikson was blonde-haired and blue-eyed, which meant he was taunted by Jews for looking Aryan and by Germans for being Jewish (Burns and Burns-Lundgren 2015). This sense of being the outsider gave him an intuitive understanding about how people belong in groups and what it takes to navigate an internal and external landscape. In the USA, he found the freedom to think differently about how we develop psychodynamically and socially.

Sigmund Freud (1856–1939)

Freud was Jewish, lived most of his life in Vienna and grew up in a complex family system. His mother, Amalia, married his father, Jakob, when she was 19 and he was 40; she was his second or third wife (the records are ambiguous). Amalia was two years older than one step-son, Emmanuel, and one year younger than her other step-son, Philipp (these dates may differ by one or two years as the records are contradictory). His step-brothers lived in the same village and had children of their own, so Freud spent time playing with his niece and nephew despite being their uncle.

Confusion and contradiction surrounded the family. Jakob was a trader selling cloth, but despite big ambitions was never successful, only just keeping his family afloat financially. Freud spent his first years in a rented single room above a blacksmith's shop. In this room, the whole of life was to be experienced, including sex, birth, and death. His devoutly Catholic nanny, who he later recalls as being his teacher in sexual matters, greatly influenced him. She was dismissed for theft but all Freud remembers is her sudden absence from his childhood world and a profound sense of loss. Out of this confusion, Freud sought certainty and security. He sought this by training as a doctor, later beginning his career as a neurologist, studying brain anatomy and function. The idea that all brain activity comes about because of connections or disconnections between what he called 'neurons' trained his thinking to focus on how things connect, and what can connect them. He understood neurons to be stimulated by essential needs, such as hunger, respiration, or sexuality, which Freud believed became instincts (1895). His thinking was influenced by Darwinian evolutionary thought and the determinist principles of nineteenth-century science.

Freud's early experience of observing the work of the famous French neurologist Charcot in Paris, and his career in private practice as a neurologist and psychological investigator, led Freud to see a series of female patients presenting with hysterical symptoms. He and a colleague, Breuer, wrote up these medical cases, which reveal his growing understanding of the power and working of the mind (Freud and Breuer 1893). Freud observed symptoms, but by listening to their personal history he discovered unspoken, censored thoughts and feelings the person had when the symptoms first appeared. Putting these into words, offering meaning through language, led to a cathartic release and a reduction of the effect of the troubling symptoms.

The next stage in Freud's development of psychoanalysis came through interpreting his dreams. He found a way of understanding and accessing the unconscious, made famous by *The Interpretation of Dreams* (1900). Many works followed including a controversial understanding of sexuality but he attracted followers including Jung. He invented the Oedipus complex to explain children's sexual and emotional development. He began an international movement as his ideas spread across Europe and to the USA. Suffering through the deaths of family and friends marked his later years, including being diagnosed with cancer of the jaw in 1923. In 1938, he left Vienna (now in Nazi control) for England. He died just before the outbreak of the Second World War and his home in Hampstead is now the Freud Museum London.

He never said, 'A cigar is just a cigar', but he did smoke them his entire life.

Carl Jung (1875–1961)

Born in Switzerland, Jung had a troubled family; his father lost his faith as a minister of religion, and his mother, who had mental health problems, believed spirits visited her at night. His personal history of precocious intelligence and solitariness led him to live in his own world, shaped from an early age by a deep engagement with mythology, the paranormal, and religious and Eastern thought.

He trained as a doctor, specialising in psychiatry at the pioneering Burghölzli Hospital in Zurich. He developed a word association test that supported the idea of unconscious processes. After meeting Freud, they developed a close relationship where Freud saw Jung as the crown prince of psychoanalysis. Freud came to see Jung as a threat to psychoanalysis because of different views around sexuality, and they parted acrimoniously. Following an intensive self-analysis from 1913 to 1917, Jung established 'analytical psychology', introducing innovative concepts including: the collective unconscious; archetypes; complexes; persona; shadow; individuation; animus; and anima (Samuels 1985). Jung saw the unconscious in more dynamic terms than Freud, including a connection beyond the self, seen in the artwork and mandalas found in *The Red Book* (2009). Based in Zurich, he travelled widely, presenting his ideas across Europe, in England, the USA, Africa, and India where he expanded his interest in the philosophy of Eastern religions.

Jung's personal life was complex, involving affairs with patients and a long-term mistress. The 1930s were controversial because of Jung's presidency of the International General Medical Society for Psychotherapy, whose German section was associated with the policies of the Nazi Party. This has led to the accusation that he was anti-Semitic and a Nazi sympathiser, an issue still hotly debated.

He continued to expand his thinking, embracing other religions, theology, and science resulting in honorary doctorates from Harvard and Oxford Universities. Jung retired in 1953 and focused on writing, including the editing of his definitive ideas published in *Collected Works* (1953–1979). His most popular book, which introduced many people to Jung for the first time, was *Memories, Dreams and Reflections* (1963), although the veracity of some of this text has been questioned.

Melanie Klein (1882–1969)

Born in Vienna in 1882, Klein was part of a large Jewish family. Hers is a story of countless struggles, domineering and ruthless figures, depression, and many deaths. Her father died in 1900 and her beloved brother Emanuel in 1902, aged 25, an immense loss as he was the one person that believed in her and supported her ambition to be a doctor. She married in 1903 to escape a domineering mother but it was an unhappy marriage, and Klein felt trapped by this traditional role and burdened in being a mother of three with Melitta born in 1904, Hans in 1907, and Eric in 1914. The family moved to Budapest and Klein tried to pursue a training in medicine, at the same time discovering the work of Freud. From 1912 to 1919, she was analysed by Ferenczi, and by 1921 read her first paper to the Hungarian Psychoanalytic Society, *The Development of a Child* (Klein 1923).

Karl Abraham, one of the pioneers of psychoanalysis, invited her to Berlin to develop this work. The move to Berlin to go into analysis with Abraham signalled the end of her disastrous and depressing marriage. She divorced in 1924, which involved a bitter dispute over custody of the children. Showing promise and original thought, Klein worked with children. Her observations revealed rich and dramatic fears and phantasies (her term) played out in the inner world of a child. In 1925, she was invited to London to give lectures on child analysis, something Ernest Jones was keen to develop. Jones was a hugely influential figure as President of the British Psychoanalytic Society, President of the International Psychoanalytic Association (1920–1924), and founder and editor of the *International Journal of Psychoanalysis*.

In 1926, Klein moved to London, where she remained for the rest of her life, and where she was to become a central figure in British psychoanalysis, one who still influences people today (Grosskurth 1986; Sayers 1991). Building on Freud's idea of drives, Klein developed new ideas and techniques including projective identification, the paranoid-schizoid position, and the depressive position. This led to conflict with Anna Freud from 1941 to 1945 in what was called the 'Controversial Discussions'. Klein's daughter, Melitta, was also a psychoanalyst in Britain but bitterly opposed her mother in these discussions. The on-going debates were so fierce that on one occasion Winnicott, who was chairing the meeting, had to remind them that the air-raid sirens were warning them of imminent bombing so it would be better to go to the air-raid shelter.

Kleinian ideas and practices found fertile ground in Britain and became the dominant model over the coming decades evolving into Post-Kleinian thought.

Jacques Lacan (1901–1981)

A French philosopher and psychoanalyst, Lacan has ever been a divider of opinions, some seeing him as a genius, others as a fraud (Forrester 1990; Fink 2017). He first emerged to prominence in the 1930s, when he argued the ego and the self emerge through our identifications with others, just as a mirror captures the image of the self and others, enabling the formation of a Subject. Lacan immersed himself in Freud's writing and the philosophy of Heidegger, Derrida, and Merleau-Ponty (to name a few). As part of the French avant-garde intellectual circle and his public seminars in 1951, he attracted a wide circle of students, academics, literary figures, and analysts. His revolutionary ideas and clinical techniques were opposed by Anna Freud and led to expulsion from the IPA (International Psychoanalytical Association). He continued to give his public seminars, which proved highly popular and influential if difficult to understand in the original French, and even more so in translation. Lacan's ideas have been widely taken up across a range of academic disciplines, and in the world-wide growth of Lacanian psychoanalysis.

Donald Woods Winnicott (1898–1971)

Born in the West Country and raised as a Methodist, Winnicott was always a non-conformist. Educated at school in Cambridge, a brief spell as a ships surgeon during the First World War led to a medical training in London. He discovered Freud and pursued training as a paediatrician and as a psychoanalyst. Winnicott qualified in medicine in 1920; married in 1923, his mother died in 1925 and his father in 1948. He worked in paediatrics at hospitals in Hackney and Paddington Green. He remained here for over 40 years, seeing an estimated 60,000 mothers and babies. Attracted to Freud's ideas, he began psychoanalysis with Strachey, who introduced him to the work of Klein. He also trained as a child psychoanalyst, supervised by Klein. During the 'Controversial Discussions' (1941–1945), he attempted to be on good terms with Anna and Klein and was part of the Independent or Middle group in the British Psychoanalytical Society.

During the Second World War, Winnicott was concerned about the psychological impact of separation on evacuees and delinquent children and he began to write, speak, and do radio talks about the importance of mothers. Through this work, he met a social worker, Clare Britton, but, prone to overwork, he had a heart attack in 1948. He recovered and married Clare in 1951, who also trained as a psychoanalyst. This became a rich period for Winnicott's writing, including six books, several more edited by Britton after his death, and a large number of papers (now available in a 12-volume *Collected Works* [2016]). Winnicott had many senior roles in British psychoanalysis and the British paediatric world. He was also influential in the IPA, with his work taken up especially in France. Winnicott survived two further heart attacks but died in 1971.

Winnicott's popular appeal lies in his use of common-sense language, as well as his evocative, poetic, and memorable phrases. His legacy is one of innovative ways of seeing how mothers and babies interact, captured with memorable phrases such as a 'good-enough mother', 'transitional objects', the 'true' and 'false' self, and 'holding', to name a few (Rodman 2003).

References

Abram, J. (2007) *The Language of Winnicott: A Dictionary of Winnicott's Use of Words*, 2nd edn. London: Karnac Books.

Abram, J. (ed.) (2013) *Donald Winnicott Today*. Hove: Routledge.

Acquarone, S. (ed.) (2016) *Surviving the Early Years: The Importance of Early Intervention with Babies at Risk*. London: Karnac Books.

Adams, M. (2010) *The Mythological Unconscious*, 2nd edn. Putnam, CT: Spring Publications.

Agassi, J. (ed.) (1999) *Martin Buber on Psychology and Psychotherapy: Essays, Letters, and Dialogue*. New York: Syracuse University Press.

Ainsworth, M. (1969) Object relations, dependency, and attachment: a theoretical review of the infant–mother relationship, *Child Development*, 40: 969–1025.

Alayarian, A. (2016) *Children of Refugees: Torture, Human Rights, and Psychological Consequences*. London: Karnac Books.

Aldridge, S. (2014) *A Short Introduction to Counselling*. London: SAGE.

Allen, J. (2013) *Restoring Mentalizing in Attachment Relationships: Treating Trauma with Plain Old Therapy*. Washington, DC: American Psychiatric Publishing.

Allen, J. and Fonagy, P. (eds.) (2006) *Handbook of Mentalization-Based Treatment*. Chichester: John Wiley.

Alpert, J. (2015) Enduring mothers, enduring knowledge: on rape and history, *Contemporary Psychoanalysis*, 51(2): 296–311.

American Psychiatric Association (APA) (2013) *The Diagnostic and Statistical Manual of Mental Disorders (DSM-5)*. Washington, DC: American Psychiatric Association.

Amis, K. (2017) *Boundaries, Power and Ethical Responsibility in Counselling and Psychotherapy*. London: SAGE.

Anzieu, D. (1989) *The Skin-Ego: A Psychoanalytic Approach to the Self*. New Haven, CT: Yale University Press.

Arean, P. and Kraemer, H. (2013) *High Quality Psychotherapy Research: From Conception to Piloting to National Trials*. Oxford: Oxford University Press.

Atwood, G. and Stolorow, R. (1984) *Structures of Subjectivity: Explorations in Psychoanalytic Phenomenology*. Hillsdale, NJ: Analytic Press.

BACP (2018) *Ethical Framework for the Counselling Professions*. Lutterworth: BACP.

Bailly, L. (2009) *Lacan: A Beginner's Guide*. Oxford: Oneworld Publications.

Balint, M. (1958) The three areas of the mind – theoretical considerations, *International Journal of Psycho-Analysis*, 39: 328–340.

Balint, M. (1968) *The Basic Fault: Therapeutic Aspects of Regression*. London: Tavistock.

Balint, M. (1969) Trauma and object relationship, *International Journal of Psycho-Analysis*, 50: 429–435.

Bambling, M., King, R., Raue, P., Schweitzer, R. and Lambert, W. (2006) Clinical supervision: its influence on client-rated working alliance and client symptom reduction in the brief treatment of major depression, *Psychotherapy Research*, 16(3): 317–331.

Barden, N. (2006) Psychodynamic counselling and gender, in S. Wheeler (ed.) *Difference and Diversity in Counselling – Contemporary Psychodynamic Practice* (pp. 39–56). Basingstoke: Palgrave Macmillan.

Barden, N. (2015) Gender, sexuality and psychoanalysis: re-evaluating Oedipal theory. Unpublished PhD thesis, University of Leicester.

Bargh, J. and Morsella, E. (2008) The unconscious mind, *Perspectives on Psychological Science*, 3(1): 73–79.

Barkham, M., Guthre, E., Hardy, G. and Margison, F. (eds.) (2016) *Psychodynamic-Interpersonal Therapy: A Conversational Model*. London: SAGE.

Barsness, R. (ed.) (2018) *Core Competencies of Relational Psychoanalysis*. Abingdon: Routledge.

Barsness, R. and Strawn, B. (2018) Relational psychoanalytic ethics, in R. Barnsness (ed.) *Core Competencies of Relational Psychoanalysis* (pp. 221–240). Abingdon: Routledge.

Bateman, A. and Fonagy, P. (2004) *Psychotherapy for Borderline Personality Disorder: Mentalisation-Based Treatment*. Oxford: Oxford University Press.

Bateman, A. and Fonagy, P. (2008) Eight-year follow-up of patients treated for borderline personality disorder: mentalization-based treatment versus treatment as usual, *American Journal of Psychiatry*, 165: 631–638.

Bateman, A. and Fonagy, P. (2009) Randomized controlled trial of outpatient mentalization-based treatment versus structured clinical management for borderline personality disorder, *American Journal of Psychiatry*, 166: 1355–1364.

Bateman, A. and Fonagy, P. (eds.) (2011) *Handbook of Mentalizing in Mental Health Practice*. Washington, DC: American Psychiatric Publishing.

Bateman, A. and Fonagy, P. (2016) *Mentalization-Based Treatment for Personality Disorders: A Practical Guide*. Oxford: Oxford University Press.

Bateman, A. and Fonagy, P. (2018) A randomized controlled trial of a mentalization-based intervention (MBT-FACTS) for families of people with borderline personality disorder, *Personality Disorders: Theory, Research, and Treatment* [DOI: 10.1037/per0000298].

BCPSG (Boston Change Process Study Group) (2010) *Change in Psychotherapy: A Unifying Paradigm*. New York: W.W. Norton.

Beebe, B. (2000) Co-constructing mother–infant distress: the microsynchrony of maternal impingement and infant avoidance in the face-to-face encounter, *Psychoanalytic Inquiry*, 20(3): 421–440.

Beebe, B. (2014) My journey in infant research and psychoanalysis: microanalysis, a social microscope, *Psychoanalytic Psychology*, 31(1): 4–25.

Beebe, B., Cohen, P. and Lachmann, F. (2016) *The Mother–Infant Interaction Picture Book*. New York: W.W. Norton.

Beebe, B., Knoblauch, S., Rustin, J., Sorter, D., Jacobs, T. and Pally, R. (2005) *Forms of Intersubjectivity in Infant Research and Adult Treatment*. New York: Other Press.

Beebe, B. and Lachmann, F. (2002) *Infant Research and Adult Treatment: Co-constructing Interactions*. Hillsdale, NJ: Analytic Press.

Beebe, B. and Lachmann, F. (2014) *The Origins of Attachment: Infant Research and Adult Treatment*. New York: Routledge.

Beebe, B. and Stern, D. (1977) Engagement–disengagement and early object experiences, in N. Freedman and S. Grand (eds.) *Communicative Structures and Psychic Structures* (pp. 35–55). New York: Plenum Press.

Benjamin, J. (1988) *The Bonds of Love: Psychoanalysis, Feminism, and the Problem of Domination*. New York: Pantheon.

Benjamin, J. (1995) *Like Subjects, Love Objects: Essays on Recognition and Sexual Difference*. New Haven, CT: Yale University Press.

Benjamin, J. (1998) *Shadow of the Other: Intersubjectivity and Gender in Psychoanalysis.* New York: Routledge.

Benjamin, J. (2004) Beyond doer and done to: an intersubjective view of thirdness, *Psychoanalytic Quarterly,* 63: 5–46.

Benjamin, J. (2013) The bonds of love: looking backward, *Studies in Gender and Sexuality,* 14(1): 1–15.

Benjamin, J. (2017) *Beyond Doer and Done To: Recognition Theory, Intersubjectivity and the Third.* New York: Routledge.

Bettelheim, B. (1982) *Freud and Man's Soul.* New York: Knopf.

Bick, E. (1968) The experience of skin in early object-relations, *International Journal of Psychoanalysis,* 49: 484–486.

Bion, W. (1961) *Experiences in Groups.* London: Tavistock.

Bion, W. (1970) *Attention and Interpretation.* London: Tavistock.

Bion, W. (1990) *Brazilian Lectures.* London: Karnac Books.

Black, D. (2011) *Why Things Matter: The Place of Values in Science, Psychoanalysis and Religion.* Hove: Routledge.

Blass, R. and Carmelli, Z. (2007) The case against neuropsychoanalysis: on fallacies underlying psychoanalysis' latest scientific trend and its negative impact on psychoanalytic discourse, *International Journal of Psychoanalysis,* 88: 19–40.

Blechner, M. (2011) Listening to the body and feeling the mind, *Contemporary Psychoanalysis,* 47(1): 25–34.

Bollas, C. (1987) *The Shadow of the Object: Psychoanalysis of the Unthought Known.* London: Routledge.

Bollas, C. (1989) *Forces of Destiny: Psychoanalysis and Human Idiom.* London: Free Association Books.

Bollas, C. (1992) *Being a Character: Psychoanalysis and Self Experience.* London: Routledge.

Bollas, C. (1999) *The Mystery of Things.* London: Routledge.

Bollas, C. (2007) *The Freudian Moment.* London: Karnac Books.

Bollas, C. (2009) *The Infinite Question.* Hove: Routledge.

Bond, T. (2018) *Ethical Framework for the Counselling Professions.* Lutterworth: BACP.

Bondi, L. and Fewell, J. (2016) *Practitioner Research in Counselling and Psychotherapy: The Power of Examples.* Basingstoke: Palgrave Macmillan.

Bordin, E.S. (1979) The generalizability of the psychoanalytic concept of the working alliance, *Psychotherapy: Theory, Research and Practice,* 16(3): 252–260.

Bowlby, J. (1969) *Attachment and Loss: Vol. 1. Attachment.* London: Hogarth Press.

Bowlby, J. (1973) *Attachment and Loss: Vol. 2. Separation, Anxiety and Anger.* London: Hogarth Press.

Bowlby, J. (1980) *Attachment and Loss: Vol. 3. Sadness and Depression.* London: Hogarth Press.

Bowlby, J. (1988) *A Secure Base: Parent–Child Attachment and Healthy Human Development.* Abingdon: Routledge.

Bowlby, J. (1989) Psychoanalysis as a natural science, in J. Sandler (ed.) *Dimensions of Psychoanalysis* (pp. 99–121). London: Karnac Books.

Bowlby, J. and Fry, M. (1953) *Childcare and the Growth of Love.* London: Penguin.

Bråten, S. (ed.) (2007) *On Being Moved: From Mirror Neurons to Empathy.* Philadelphia, PA: John Benjamins.

Britton, R. (1998) *Belief and Imagination: Explorations in Psychoanalysis.* London: Routledge.

Britton, R., Feldman, M., O'Shaughnessy, E. and Steiner, J. (eds.) (1989) *The Oedipus Complex Today: Clinical Implications.* London: Karnac Books.

Bromberg, P. (1996) Standing in the spaces: the multiplicity of self and the psychoanalytic relationship, *Contemporary Psychoanalysis,* 32: 509–535.

Bromberg, P. (2001) *Standing in the Spaces: Essays on Clinical Process, Trauma and Dissociation.* Hillsdale, NJ: Analytic Press.

Bromberg, P. (2006) *Awakening the Dreamer: Clinical Journeys.* Hillsdale, NJ: Analytic Press.

Brothers, D. (2014) Traumatic attachments: intergenerational trauma, dissociation, and the analytic relationship, *International Journal of Psychoanalytic Self Psychololgy*, 9(1): 3–15.

Brunner, J. (1991) Psychiatry, psychoanalysis, and politics during the First World War, *Journal of the History of Behavioural Sciences*, 27: 352–364.

Bruschweiler-Stern, N. (2009) Moments of meeting: pivotal moments in mother, infant, father bonding: Switzerland, in K. Nugent, B. Petrauskis and T. Brazelton (eds.) *The Newborn as a Person: Enabling Healthy Infant Development World-Wide* (pp. 70–84). Hoboken, NJ: John Wiley.

Buber, M. (1958) *I and Thou* (trans. R.G. Smith). New York: Charles Scribner's Sons.

Burns, T. and Burns-Lundgren, E. (2015) *Psychotherapy: A Very Short Introduction.* Oxford: Oxford University Press.

Byrne, D. (1998) *Complexity Theory and the Social Sciences.* London: Routledge.

Cabaniss, D., Cherry, S., Douglas, C. and Schwartz, A. (2011) *Psychodynamic Psychotherapy: A Clinical Manual.* Chichester: John Wiley.

Caldwell, L. and Joyce, A. (eds.) (2011) *Reading Winnicott.* Hove: Routledge.

Casement, P. (1985) *On Learning from the Patient.* London: Routledge.

Casement, P. (1990) *Further Learning from the Patient: The Analytic Space and Process.* London: Tavistock/Routledge.

Casement, P. (2002) *Learning from Our Mistakes: Beyond Dogma in Psychoanalysis and Psychotherapy.* New York: Guilford Press.

Castonguay, L. and Oltmanns, T. (eds.) (2013) *Psychopathology: From Science to Clinical Practice.* New York: Guilford Press.

Chodorow, N. (1989) *Feminism and Psychoanalytic Theory.* New Haven, CT: Yale University Press.

Clare, A. and Thompson, S. (1981) *Let's Talk About Me: A Critical Examination of the New Psychotherapies.* London: British Broadcasting Corporation.

Clarke, J. (2018) Guest editorial, *Psychoanalytic Psychotherapy*, 32(2): 95–101.

Coates, S. (2004) John Bowlby and Margaret S. Mahler: their lives and theories, *Journal of the American Psychoanalytic Association*, 52(2): 571–601.

Coltart, N. (1992) *Slouching Towards Bethlehem: And Further Psychoanalytic Explorations.* London: Free Association Books.

Cook, R., Bird, G., Catmur, C., Press, C. and Heyes, C. (2014) Mirror neurons: from origin to function, *Behavioural and Brain Sciences*, 37: 177–241.

Cooper, M. (2008) *Essential Research Findings in Counselling and Psychotherapy.* London: SAGE.

Coren, A. (2010) *Short-term Psychotherapy: A Psychodynamic Approach*, 2nd edn. Basingstoke: Palgrave.

Coren, A. (2016) Short-term therapy: therapy-lite?, in D. Mair (ed.) *Short-Term Counselling in Higher Education: Context, Theory and Practice* (pp. 29–44). Abingdon: Routledge.

Cornish, J. (2009) *Scotland's Mountains.* London: Aurum Press.

Cozolino, L. (2016) *Why Therapy Works: Using Our Minds to Change Our Brains.* New York: W.W. Norton.

Dalal, F. (1998) *Taking the Group Seriously: Towards a Post-Foulkesian Group Analytic Theory.* London: Jessica Kingsley.

Dalal, F. (2011) The social unconscious and ideology in clinical theory and practice, in E. Hopper and H. Weinberg (eds.) *The Social Unconscious in Persons, Groups, and Societies* (pp. 243–263). London: Karnac Books.

Damasio, A. (2012) *Self Comes to Mind: Constructing the Conscious Brain.* London: Vintage.

Danchev, A. (1998) *Alchemist of War: The Life of Basil Liddel Hart.* London: Weidenfeld & Nicolson.

Danchev, A. (2012) *Cezanne: A Life.* London: Profile Books.

Danchev, D. and Ross, A. (2013) *Research Ethics for Counsellors, Nurses and Social Workers*. London: SAGE.

Daniel, S. (2006) Adult attachment patterns and individual psychotherapy: a review, *Clinical Psychology Review*, 26: 968–984.

Davey, G. (2014) *Psychopathology: Research, Assessment and Treatment in Clinical Psychology*, 2nd edn. Chichester: John Wiley.

Davies, J. (2011) *The Importance of Suffering: The Value and Meaning of Emotional Discontent*. Hove: Routledge.

Davies, J. (2014) *Cracked: Why Psychiatry is Doing More Harm than Good*. London: Icon Books.

Deleuze, G. and Guattari, F. [1972] (1983 English trans.) *Anti-Oedipus: Capitalism and Schizophrenia*. London: Athlone Press.

Dicks, H. (1970) *Fifty Years of the Tavistock Clinic*. London: Routledge & Kegan Paul.

Dimen, M. and Goldner, V. (2012) Gender and sexuality, in G. Gabbard, B. Litowitz and P. Williams (eds.) *Textbook of Psychoanalysis*, 2nd edn. (pp. 133–152). Washington, DC: American Psychiatric Publishing.

Doidge, N. (2008) *The Brain that Changes Itself: Stories of Personal Triumph from the Frontiers of Brain Science*, rev. edn. London: Penguin Books.

Edgcumbe, R. (2000) *Anna Freud: A View of Development, Disturbance and Therapeutic Techniques*. London: Routledge.

Ehrenberg, D. (1974) The intimate edge in therapeutic relatedness, *Contemporary Psychoanalysis*, 10: 423–437.

Ehrenberg, D. (1992) *The Intimate Edge*. New York: W.W. Norton.

Eigen, M. (1981) The area of faith in Winnicott, Lacan and Bion, *International Journal of Psychoanalysis*, 62: 413–433.

Eigen, M. (1998) *The Psychoanalytic Mystic*. London: Free Association Books.

Eigen, M. (2012) *Psychoanalysis and Kabbalah*. London: Karanc Books.

Eigen, M. (2014) *A Felt Sense: More Explorations of Psychoanalysis and Kabbalah*. London: Karanc Books.

Eleftheriadou, Z. (2016) Creating a safe space: psychotherapeutic support for refugee parents and babies, in S. Acquarone (ed.) *Surviving the Early Years: The Importance of Early Intervention with Babies at Risk* (pp. 87–99). London: Karnac Books.

Ellenberger, H. (1970) *The Discovery of the Unconscious: The History and Evolution of Dynamic Psychiatry*. New York: Basic Books.

Emde, R. (2013) Remembering Daniel Stern (1934–2012): a legacy for 21st century psychoanalytic thinking and practice, *International Journal of Psychoanalysis*, 94(4): 857–861.

Erikson, E. (1950) *Childhood and Society*. New York: W.W. Norton.

Erikson, E. (1959) *Identity and the Life Cycle*. New York: International Universities Press.

Fairbairn, W.R.D. (1944) *Psychoanalytic Studies of the Personality*. London: Routledge & Kegan Paul.

Falzeder, E. (2012) Freud and Jung, Freudians and Jungians, *Jung Journal: Culture and Psyche*, 6(3): 24–43.

Fear, R. (2015) *The Oedipus Complex: Solutions or Resolutions?* London: Karnac Books.

Ferrari, P. and Rizzolatti, G. (2014) Mirror neuron research: the past and the future, *Philosophical Transactions of the Royal Society B: Biological Sciences*, 369(1644): 20130169.

Field, N. (1989). Listening with the body: an exploration in the countertransference, *British Journal of Psychotherapy*, 5(4): 512–522.

Fink, B. (1997) *A Clinical Introduction to Lacanian Psychoanalysis: Theory and Technique*. Cambridge, MA: Harvard University Press.

Fink, B. (2017) *A Clinical Introduction to Freud: Techniques for Everyday Practice*. New York: W.W. Norton.

Finlay, L. (2016) *Relational Integrative Psychotherapy: Engaging Process and Theory in Practice*. Chichester: Wiley-Blackwell.

Fjeldstad, A., Höglend, P. and Lorentzen, S. (2016) Presence of personality disorder moderates the long-term effects of short-term and long-term psychodynamic group therapy: a 7-year follow-up of a randomized clinical trial, *Group Dynamics: Theory, Research, and Practice*, 20(4): 294–309.

Fletcher, J. (2013) *Freud and the Scene of Trauma*. New York: Fordham University Press.

Fletcher, J. and Ray, N. (eds.) (2014) *Seductions and Enigmas: Laplanche, Theory, Culture*. London: Lawrence & Wishart.

Fonagy, P. (2001) *Attachment Theory and Psychoanalysis*. New York: Other Press.

Fonagy, P. (2010) Psychotherapy research: do we know what works for whom?, *British Journal of Psychiatry*, 197(2): 83–85.

Fonagy, P. (2015) The effectiveness of psychodynamic psychotherapies: an update, *World Psychiatry*, 14(2): 137–150.

Fonagy, P., Cotterell, D., Phillips, J., Bevington, D., Glaser, D. and Allison, E. (2016) *What Works for Whom? A Critical Review of Treatments for Children and Adolescents*, 2nd edn. New York: Guilford Press.

Fonagy, P., Gergely, G., Jurist, E. and Target, M. (2004) *Affect Regulation, Mentalization, and the Development of the Self*. New York: Other Press.

Fonagy, P., Kächele, H., Leuzinger-Bohleber, M. and Taylor, D. (eds.) (2012) *The Significance of Dreams: Bridging Clinical and Extraclinical Research in Psychoanalysis*. London: Karnac Books.

Fonagy, P., Leuzinger-Bohleber, M. and Krause, R. (eds.) (2009) *Identity, Gender, and Sexuality: 150 Years After Freud*. London: Karnac Books.

Fonagy, P. and Target, M. (1996) Predictors of outcome in child psychoanalysis: a retrospective study of 763 cases at the Anna Freud Centre, *Journal of the American Psychoanalytic Association*, 44: 27–77.

Fonagy, P. and Target, M. (2003) *Psychoanalytic Theories: Perspectives from Developmental Psychopathology*. London: Whurr Publishers.

Fonagy, P. and Target, M. (2007) The rooting of the mind in the body: new links between attachment theory and psychoanalytic thought, *Journal of the American Psychoanalytic Association*, 55(2): 411–456.

Forrester, J. (1990) *The Seductions of Psychoanalysis: Essays on Freud, Lacan, and Derrida*. Cambridge: Cambridge University Press.

Foulkes, S.H. (1964) *Therapeutic Group Analysis*. London: George Allen & Unwin.

Frawley-O'Dea, M. and Sarnat, J. (2001) *The Supervisory Relationship: A Contemporary Psychodynamic Approach*. New York: Guilford Press.

Freud, A. (1936) *The Ego and the Mechanisms of Defence*. London: Hogarth Press.

Freud, A. (1960) Discussion of Dr. John Bowlby's paper, *Psychoanalytic Study of the Child*, 15: 53–62.

Freud, A. (1963) The concept of developmental lines, *Psychoanalytic Study of the Child*, 18: 245–265.

Freud, A. (1981) The concept of developmental lines – their diagnostic significance, *Psychoanalytic Study of the Child*, 36: 129–136.

Note: Freud's writings were published as *The Standard Edition of the Complete Psychological Works of Sigmund Freud*. London: Hogarth Press. I adopt the standard abbreviation *S.E.* and the date the papers were originally published.

Freud, S. (and Breuer, J.) (1893–1895) Studies on Hysteria, *S.E.* (Vol. 2).

Freud, S. (1894) The Neuro-Psychoses of Defence, *S.E.* (Vol. 3, pp. 41–61).

Freud, S. (1895) Project for a Scientific Psychology, *S.E.* (Vol. 3, pp. 283–397).

Freud, S. (1896) Further Remarks on the Neuro-Psychoses of Defence, *S.E.* (Vol. 3, pp. 157–185).

Freud, S. (1900a) The Interpretation of Dreams (First Part), *S.E.* (Vol. 4).

Freud, S. (1900b) The Interpretation of Dreams (Second Part), *S.E.* (Vol. 5).

Freud, S. (1901) The Psychopathology of Everyday Life, *S.E.* (Vol. 6).

Freud, S. (1905a) Three Essays on the Theory of Sexuality, *S.E.* (Vol. 7, pp. 123–246).

Freud, S. (1905b) On Psychotherapy, *S.E.* (Vol. 7, pp. 256–268).

Freud, S. (1905c) Fragment of an Analysis of a Case of Hysteria, *S.E.* (Vol. 7, pp. 1–122).

Freud, S. (1908) Creative Writers and Day-Dreaming, *S.E.* (Vol. 9, pp. 141–154).

Freud, S. (1909) Analysis of a Phobia in a Five-year-old Boy, *S.E.* (Vol. 10, pp. 3–149).

Freud, S. (1910) Five Lectures on Psychoanalysis, *S.E.* (Vol. 11, pp. 3–56).

Freud, S. (1913) On Beginning the Treatment, *S.E.* (Vol. 12, pp. 123–144).

Freud, S. (1914a) On the History of the Psycho-Analytic Movement, *S.E.* (Vol. 14, pp. 7–66).

Freud, S. (1914b) Remembering, Repeating and Working-Through, *S.E.* (Vol. 12, pp. 145–156).

Freud, S. (1915a) Repression, *S.E.* (Vol. 14, pp. 141–158).

Freud, S. (1915b) The Unconscious, *S.E.* (Vol. 14, pp. 159–215).

Freud, S. (1920) Beyond the Pleasure Principle, *S.E.* (Vol. 19, pp. 1–64).

Freud, S. (1923) The Ego and the Id, *S.E.* (Vol. 19, pp. 3–63).

Freud, S. (1927) The Future of an Illusion, *S.E.* (Vol. 21, pp. 3–56).

Freud, S. (1930) Civilization and Its Discontents, *S.E.* (Vol. 21, pp. 57–146).

Freud, S. (1937) Analysis Terminable and Interminable, *S.E.* (Vol. 23, pp. 216–253).

Freud, S. (1938) The Technique of Psychoanalysis, *S.E.* (Vol. 23, pp. 172–182).

Freud, S. and Freud, A. (2014) *Correspondence of Sigmund Freud and Anna Freud 1904–1938.* Cambridge: Polity Press.

Friedländer, S. (2007) *The Years of Extermination: Nazi Germany and the Jews 1939–1945.* New York: HarperCollins.

Friedman, R. (2009) The issue of homosexuality in psychoanalysis, in P. Fonagy and M. Leuzinger-Bohleber (eds.) *Identity, Gender, and Sexuality: 150 Years After Freud* (pp. 79–97). London: Karnac Books.

Gabbard, G. (2010) *Long-Term Psychodynamic Psychotherapy: A Basic Text,* 2nd edn. Washington, DC: American Psychiatric Publishing.

Gabbard, G. (2016) *Boundaries and Boundary Violations in Psychoanalysis,* 2nd edn. Washington, DC: American Psychiatric Publishing.

Gallese, V. (2003) The roots of empathy: the shared manifold hypothesis and the neural basis of inter-subjectivity, *Psychopathology,* 36(4): 171–180.

Gallese, V., Eagle, M. and Migone, P. (2007) Intentional attunement: mirror neurons and the neural underpinnings of interpersonal relations, *Journal of the American Psychoanalytic Association,* 55(1): 131–175.

Gay, P. (1998) *Freud: A Life for Our Time,* 2nd edn. New York: W.W. Norton.

Gazzillo, F., Schimmenti, A., Formica, I., Simonelli, A. and Salvatore, S. (2017) Effectiveness is the gold standard of clinical research, *Research in Psychotherapy: Psychopathology, Process and Outcome,* 20: 153–155.

Geller, J., Norcross, J. and Orlinsky, D. (eds.) (2005) *The Psychotherapist's Own Psychotherapy: Patient and Clinician Perspectives.* New York: Oxford University Press.

Gerhardt, S. (2015) *Why Love Matters: How Affection Shapes a Baby's Brain,* 2nd edn. Hove: Routledge.

Gerson, S. (2004) The relational unconscious: a core element of intersubjectivity, thirdness, and clinical process, *Psychoanalytic Quarterly,* 73(1): 63–98.

Gildea, R. (2015) *Fighters in the Shadows: A New History of the French Resistance.* London: Faber & Faber.

Gilmore, K. (2012) Childhood experiences and the adult world, in G. Gabbard, B. Litowitz and P. Williams (eds.) *Textbook of Psychoanalysis,* 2nd edn. (pp. 117–131). Washington, DC: American Psychiatric Publishing.

Ginot, E. (2015) *The Neuropsychology of the Unconscious: Integrating Brain and Mind in Psychotherapy.* New York: W.W. Norton.

Gipps, R. (2013) Cognitive behaviour therapy: a philosophical appraisal, in K.W.M. Fulford, M. Davies, R. Gipps, G. Graham, J. Sadler, G. Stanghellini and T. Thornton (eds.) *The Oxford Handbook of Philosophy and Psychiatry* (pp. 1245–1263). Oxford: Oxford University Press.

Golding, K. (ed.) (2007) *Attachment Theory into Practice*, Briefing Paper No. 26. Leicester: BPS.

Gomez, L. (1996) *Introduction to Object Relations.* London: Free Association Books.

Gomez, L. (2017) *Developments in Object Relations: Controversies, Conflicts, and Common Ground.* Abingdon: Routledge.

Gordon, R. (2001) MMPI/MMPI-2 changes in long–term psychoanalytic psychotherapy, *Issues in Psychoanalytic Psychology*, 23(1/2): 59–79.

Gordon, R.M. (2010) The scientific renaissance of psychodynamic therapy (PDT), *Pennsylvania Psychologist Quarterly*, 70(3): 22–23. Available at: https://www.mmpi-info.com/gordon-r-m-2010-the-scientific-ren [accessed 30 September 2017].

Gray, A. (1994) *An Introduction to the Therapeutic Frame.* London: Routledge.

Green, D. and Latchford, G. (2012) *Maximising the Benefits of Psychotherapy: A Practice-Based Evidence Approach.* Chichester: Wiley-Blackwell.

Green, V. (ed.) (2003) *Emotional Development in Psychoanalysis, Attachment Theory and Neuroscience: Creating Connections.* Hove: Brunner-Routledge.

Greenberg, J. (2012) Psychoanalysis in North America after Freud, in G. Gabbard, B. Litowitz and P. Williams (eds.) *Textbook of Psychoanalysis*, 2nd edn. (pp. 19–35). Washington, DC: American Psychiatric Publishing.

Grosskurth, P. (1986) *Melanie Klein: Her World and Her Work.* Northvale, NJ: Jason Aronson.

Grosz, S. (2013) *The Examined Life. How We Lose and Find Ourselves.* London: Chatto & Windus.

Grotstein, J. (2007) *A Beam of Intense Darkness: Wilfred Bion's Legacy to Psychoanalysis.* London: Karnac Books.

Guntrip, H. (1969) *Schizoid Phenomena, Object Relations, and the Self.* New York: International Universities Press.

Hart, B. (1916) *The Psychology of Insanity*, 3rd edn. Cambridge: Cambridge University Press.

Hartmann, H. (1958) *Ego Psychology and the Problem of Adaptation.* New York: International Universities Press.

Hayman, A. (1989) What do we mean by 'phantasy'?, *International Journal of Psycho-Analysis*, 70: 105–114.

Hayton, A. (ed.) (2007) *Untwinned: Perspectives on the Death of a Twin Before Birth.* St. Albans: Wren Publications.

Hazell, J. (1996) *H.J.S. Guntrip: A Psychoanalytical Biography.* London: Free Association Books.

Heard, D., Lake, B. and McCluskey, U. (2012) *Attachment Therapy with Adolescents and Adults: Theory and Practice Post Bowlby*, rev. edn. London: Karnac Books.

Hendrix, J. (2015) *Unconscious Thought in Philosophy and Psychoanalysis.* Basingstoke: Palgrave Macmillan.

Herman, J. (1992) *Trauma and Recovery.* New York: Basic Books.

Hobson, R.P. (2016) *Brief Psychoanalytic Therapy.* Oxford: Oxford University Press.

Hodson, P. (2012) *The Business of Therapy: How to Run a Successful Private Practice.* Maidenhead: Open University Press.

Hoffman, I. (1998) *Ritual and Spontaneity in the Psychoanalytic Process.* Hillsdale, NJ: Analytic Press.

Hoffman, M. (2011) *Toward Mutual Recognition: Relational Psychoanalysis and the Christian Narrative.* New York: Routledge.

Hollanders, H. (2007) Integrative and eclectic approaches, in W. Dryden (ed.) *Dryden's Handbook of Individual Therapy*, 5th edn. (pp. 424–450). London: SAGE.

Holmes, J. (2001) *The Search for the Secure Base: Attachment Theory and Psychotherapy*. London: Routledge.

Holmes, J. (2010) *Exploring in Security: Attachment-Informed Psychoanalytic Psychotherapy*. Hove: Routledge.

Holmes, J. (2014) *John Bowlby and Attachment Theory*, 2nd edn. Hove: Routledge.

Holmes, J. and Bateman, A. (eds.) (2002) *Integration in Psychotherapy: Models and Methods*. Oxford: Oxford University Press.

Hooker, C., Verosky, S., Germine, L., Knight, R. and D'Esposito, M. (2008) Mentalizing about emotion and its relationship to empathy, *Social Cognitive and Affective Neuroscience*, 3(3): 204–217.

Hopper, E. (1996) The social unconscious in clinical work, *Group*, 20(1): 7–42.

Hopper, E. (2001) The social unconscious: theoretical considerations, *Group Analysis*, 34(1): 9–27.

Hopper, E. (2003) *Traumatic Experience in the Unconscious Life of Groups*. London: Jessica Kingsley.

Horvath, A. and Greenberg, L. (1989) Development and validation of the Working Alliance Inventory, *Journal of Counseling Psychology*, 36(2): 223–233.

Howard, S. (2017) *Skills in Psychodynamic Counselling & Psychotherapy*, 2nd edn. London: SAGE.

Howell, E. and Itzkowitz, S. (eds.) (2016) *The Dissociative Mind in Psychoanalysis: Understanding and Working with Trauma*. New York: Routledge.

Jacobs, M. (1982) *Still Small Voice: A Practical Introduction to Counselling for Pastors and Other Helpers*. London: SPCK.

Jacobs, M. (1986) *The Presenting Past: An Introduction to Practical Psychodynamic Counselling*. Buckingham: Open University Press.

Jacobs, M. (1988) *Psychodynamic Counselling in Action*. London: SAGE.

Jacobs, M. (2011) The aims of personal therapy in training, *Psychodynamic Practice*, 17(4): 427–439.

Jacobs, M. (2012) *The Presenting Past: The Core of Psychodynamic Counselling and Therapy*, 4th edn. Maidenhead: Open University Press.

Jones, E. (2004) War and the practice of psychotherapy: the UK experience 1939–1960, *Medical History*, 48(4): 493–510.

Jones, G. (1999) Beyond the oedipal complex: Freud and Lacan revisited, *Psychodynamic Counselling*, 5(4): 453–463.

Joseph, B. (1985) Transference: the total situation, *International Journal of Psycho-Analysis*, 66: 447–454.

Jung, C. (1953–1979) *The Collected Works of C G. Jung*, Vols. 1–20. London: Routledge & Kegan Paul.

Jung, C. [1933] (1964) *The Collected Works of C.G. Jung*, Vol. 10. London: Routledge & Kegan Paul.

Jung, C. (1977) *Memories, Dreams, Reflections*. Glasgow: Collins/Fountain Books.

Jung, C. (2009) *The Red Book: Liber Novus*. New York: W.W. Norton.

Kahr, B. (2016) *Tea with Winnicott*. London: Karnac Books.

Kalsched, D. (2003) Daimonic elements in early trauma, *Journal of Analytic Psychology*, 48(2): 145–169.

Kalsched, D. (2013) *Trauma and the Soul: A Psycho-Spiritual Approach to Human Development and its Interruption*. Hove: Routledge.

Kenny, D. (2013) *Bringing Up Baby: The Psychoanalytic Infant Comes of Age*. London: Karnac Books.

Kenny, D. (2015) *God, Freud and Religion: The Origins of Faith, Fear and Fundamentalism*. Hove: Routledge.

Khan, M. (1963) The concept of cumulative trauma, *Psychoanalytic Study of the Child*, 18: 286–306.

King, M.L., Jr. (1968) Available at: https://kinginstitute.stanford.edu/king-papers/publications/knock-midnight-inspiration-great-sermons-reverend-martin-luther-king-jr-10 [accessed 9 January 2019].

King, P. and Steiner, R. (eds.) (1992) *The Freud–Klein Controversies 1941–1945*. London: Routledge.

Kirsner, D. (2000) *Unfree Associations: Inside Psychoanalytic Institutes*. London: Process Press.

Klein, M. (1923) The development of a child, *International Journal of Psychoanalysis*, 4: 419–474.

Kohon, G. (ed.) (1986) *The British School of Psychoanalysis: The Independent Tradition*. London: Free Association Books.

Kohut, H. (1977) *The Restoration of the Self*. New York: International Universities Press.

Kollias, H. (2009) Psychoanalysis and philosophy, in J. Mullarkey and B. Lord (eds.) *The Bloomsbury Companion to Continental Philosophy* (pp. 145–165). London: Bloomsbury Publishing.

Krause-Utz, A., Winter, D., Niedtfeld, I. and Schmahl, C. (2014) The latest neuroimaging findings in borderline personality disorder, *Current Psychiatry Reports*, 16(3): 438.

Kuhn, P. (2016) *Psychoanalysis in Britain, 1893–1913: Histories and Historiography*. Lanham, MD: Lexington Books.

Kuhn, T. (2012) *The Structures of Scientific Revolutions*, 50th anniversary edn. Chicago, IL: University of Chicago Press.

Kwawer, J. (1998) On using Winnicott, *Contemporary Psychoanalysis*, 34(3): 389–395.

Lacan, J. (1977) *The Four Fundamental Concepts of Psychoanalysis*. London: Hogarth Press.

Lacewing, M. (2013) Could psychoanalysis be a science, in K.W.M. Fulford, M. Davies, R. Gipps, G. Graham, J. Sadler, G. Stanghellini and T. Thornton (eds.) *The Oxford Handbook of Philosophy and Psychiatry* (pp. 1103–1127). Oxford: Oxford University Press.

Lake, F. (1966) *Clinical Theology: A Theological and Psychiatric Basis to Clinical Pastoral Care*. London: DLT.

Laplanche, J. (1987) *New Foundations for Psychoanalysis* (trans. Jonathan House, 2016). New York: The Unconscious in Translation.

Lapanche, J. and Pontalis, J.B. (1973) *The Language of Psycho-Analysis*. London: Hogarth Press.

Lawrence, D.H. (1921) *Psychoanalysis and the Unconscious*. New York: Thomas Seltzer.

Lear, J. (2015) *Freud*, 2nd edn. Abingdon: Routledge.

Lee, R. (1968) *Principles of Pastoral Counselling*. London: SPCK.

Leighton, J. (2007) Enhancing psychoanalysis: a case of integrating EMDR, *Psychoanalytic Perspectives*, 5(1): 105–125.

Leiper, R. with Kent, R. (2001) *Working Through Setbacks in Psychotherapy: Crisis, Impasse and Relapse*. London: SAGE.

Leiper, R. (2014) Psychodynamic formulation: looking below the surface, in L. Johnstone and R. Dallos (eds.) *Formulation in Psychology and Psychotherapy*, 2nd edn. (pp. 45–66). Hove: Routledge.

Lemma, A. (2010) *Under the Skin: A Psychoanalytic Study of Body Modification*. Hove: Routledge.

Lemma, A. (2012) Research off the couch: re-visiting the transsexual conundrum, *Psychoanalytic Psychotherapy*, 26(4): 263–281.

Lemma, A. (2013) The body one has and the body one is: understanding the transsexual's need to be seen, *International Journal of Psychoanalysis*, 94: 277–292.

Lemma, A. (2016) *Introduction to the Practice of Psychoanalytic Psychotherapy*, 2nd edn. Chichester: John Wiley & Sons.

Lemma, A. and Lynch, P. (eds.) (2015) *Sexualities: Contemporary Psychoanalytic Perspectives*. Hove: Routledge.

Lemma, A., Target, M. and Fonagy, P. (2011) *Brief Dynamic Interpersonal Therapy: A Clinician's Guide*. Oxford: Oxford University Press.

Leonoff, A. (2013) Metaphor-work in the treatment of complex psychic trauma, *Canadian Journal of Psychoanalysis*, 21(2): 247–269.

Levine, L. and Brown, L. (eds.) (2013) *Growth and Turbulence in the Container/Contained: Bion's Continuing Legacy*. Hove: Routledge.

Lewin, V. (2004) *The Twin in The Transference*. London: Whurr Publishers.

Lewis, C.S. (1956) *Till We Have Faces*. London: Geoffrey Bles.

Lewis, C.S. (1960) *The Four Loves*. London: Geoffrey Bles.

Lewis, C.S. (1961) *A Grief Observed*. London: Faber & Faber.

Likierman, M. (2002) *Melanie Klein: Her Work in Context*. London: Quantum.

Lilliengren, P. and Sköndal, E. (2017) Comprehensive Compilation of Randomized Controlled Trials (RCTs) Involving Psychodynamic Treatments and Interventions. Last updated 17 October 2017. Available at: https://www.researchgate.net/publication/317335876_Comprehensive_compilation_of_randomized_controlled_trials_RCTs_involving_psychodynamic_treatments_and_interventions [accessed 25 October 2017].

Lingiardi, V. and McWilliams, N. (eds.) (2017) *Psychodynamic Diagnostic Manual, Second Edition: (PDM–2)*. New York: Guilford Press.

Loewenberg, P. and Thompson, N. (eds.) (2011) *100 Years of the IPA: The Centenary History of the International Psychoanalytical Association 1910–2010 – Evolution and Change*. London: Karnac Books.

Long, P. and Lepper, G. (2008) Metaphor in psychoanalytic psychotherapy: a comparative study of four cases by a practitioner-researcher, *British Journal of Psychotherapy*, 24: 343–364.

Loparic, Z. (2013) From Freud to Winnicott: aspects of a paradigm change, in J. Abram (ed.) *Donald Winnicott Today* (pp. 113–156). Hove: Routledge.

López-Corvo, R.E. (2003) *The Dictionary of the Work of W.R. Bion*. London: Karnac Books.

Luxmore, N. (2016) *Horny and Hormonal: Young People, Sex and the Anxieties of Sexuality*. London: Jessica Kingsley.

Lyons-Ruth, K. (1991) Rapprochement or approchement: Mahler's theory reconsidered from the vantage point of recent research on early attachment relationships, *Psychoanalytic Psychology*, 8(1): 1–23.

Lyons-Ruth, K. (1998) Implicit relational knowing: its role in development and psychoanalytic treatment, *Infant Mental Health Journal*, 19: 282–289.

Lyons-Ruth, K. (1999) The two–person unconscious: intersubjective dialogue, enactive relational representation, and the emergence of new forms of relational organization, *Psychoanalytic Inquiry*, 19(4): 576–617.

Mahler, M., Pine, F. and Bergman, A. (1975) *The Psychological Birth of the Human Infant: Symbiosis and Individuation*. New York: Basic Books.

Main, M. and Solomon, J. (1986) Discovery of an insecure-disorganized/disoriented attachment pattern, in T.B. Brazelton and M.W. Yogman (eds.) *Affective Development in Infancy* (pp. 95–124). Westport, CT: Ablex Publishing.

Malan, D. (1979) *Individual Psychotherapy and the Science of Psychodynamics*. Oxford: Butterworth Heinemann.

Malan, D. and Coughlin Della Selva, P. (2006) *Lives Transformed: A Revolutionary Method of Dynamic Psychotherapy*. London: Karnac Books.

Mancia, M. (1981) On the beginning of mental life in the foetus, *International Journal of Psychoanalysis*, 62: 351–357.

Mancia, M. (ed.) (2006) *Psychoanalysis and Neuroscience*. Milan: Springer-Verlag.

Masson, J. (ed. and trans.) (1985) *The Complete Letters of Sigmund Freud to Wilhelm Fliess, 1887–1904*. Cambridge, MA: Harvard University Press.

Mawson, C. (ed.) (2010) *Bion Today*. London: Routledge.

May, U. (2001) Abraham's discovery of the 'bad mother': a contribution to the history of the theory of depression, *International Journal of Psychoanalysis*, 82: 283–305.

McCulloch, J. (2009) Grappling with tenderness in psychoanalysis, in B. Willock, R. Curtis and L. Bohm (eds.) *Taboo or not Taboo? Forbidden Thoughts, Forbidden Acts in Psychoanalysis and Psychotherapy* (pp. 65–74). London: Karnac Books.

McGilchrist, I. (2009) *The Master and his Emissary: The Divided Brain and the Making of the Western World*. New Haven, CT: Yale University Press.

McLeod, J. (2010) *Case Study Research in Counselling and Psychotherapy*. London: BACP/SAGE.

McLeod, J. (2016) *Using Research in Counselling and Psychotherapy*. London: SAGE.

McWilliams, N. (1999) *Psychoanalytic Case Formulation*. New York: Guilford Press.

McWilliams, N. (2004) *Psychoanalytic Therapy: A Practitioner's Guide*. New York: Guilford Press.

Meek, H. (2003) The place of the unconscious in qualitative research, *Forum Qualitative Sozialforschung/Forum: Qualitative Social Research*, 4(2). Available at: http://www.qualitative-research.net/index.php/fqs/article/view/711/1540 [accessed 15 July 2018].

Meng, H. and Freud, E. (eds.) (1963) *Psychoanalysis and Faith: The Letters of Sigmund Freud and Oskar Pfister*. New York: Basic Books.

Midgley, N. (2013) *Reading Anna Freud*. London: Routledge.

Mills, J. (2002) *The Unconscious Abyss: Hegel's Anticipation of Psychoanalysis*. Albany, NY: State University of New York Press.

Mitchell, J. (1974) *Psychoanalysis and Feminism*. New York: Pantheon.

Mitchell, J. (2003) *Siblings: Sex and Violence*. Cambridge: Polity Press.

Mitchell, M. (2009) *Complexity: A Guided Tour*. Oxford: Oxford University Press.

Mitchell, S. (1993) *Hope and Dread in Psychoanalysis*. New York: Basic Books.

Mitchell, S. (1998) From ghosts to ancestors: the psychoanalytic vision of Hans Loewald, *Psychoanalytic Dialogues*, 8(6): 825–888.

Mitchels, B. and Bond, T. (2011) Legal issues across counselling and psychotherapy *settings*. London: BACP/SAGE.

Molino, A. (ed.) (1997) *Freely Associated Encounters in Psychoanalysis with Christopher Bollas, Joyce McDougall, Michael Eigen, Adam Phillips, Nina Coltart*. London: Free Associations Books.

Mollon, P. (1996) *Multiple Selves, Multiple Voices: Working with Trauma, Violation and Dissociation*. Chichester: John Wiley.

Mollon, P. (2001) *Releasing the Self: The Healing Legacy of Heinz Kohut*. London: Whurr Publishers.

Mollon, P. (2004) *EMDR and the Energy Therapies: Psychoanalytic Perspectives*. London: Karnac Books.

Mollon, P. (2008) *Psychoanalytic Energy Psychotherapy*. London: Karnac Books.

Mollon, P. (2012) The foreclosure of disassociation in psychoanalysis, in V. Sinason (ed.) *Trauma, Dissociations and Multiplicity: Working on Identity and Selves* (pp. 8–20). Hove: Routledge.

Mollon, P. (2016) Releasing the Unknown Self. Available at: http://selfpsychologypsychoanalysis.org/mollon.shtml [accessed 1 December 2016].

Muran, C. (2007) *Dialogues on Difference: Studies of Diversity in the Therapeutic Relationship*. Washington, DC: American Psychological Association.

Murdin, L. (2009) *Understanding Transference: The Power of Patterns in the Therapeutic Relationship*. Basingstoke: Palgrave.

Murdin, L. (2015) *Managing Difficult Endings in Psychotherapy*. London: Karnac Books.

Nettleton, S. (2017) *The Metapsychology of Christopher Bollas*. Abingdon: Routledge.

Nietzsche, F. (1887) *The Gay Science*. Leipzig: E.W. Fritzsch.

Noonan, E. (2003) *Counselling Young People*. London: Methuen.

Norcross, J. (ed.) (2011) *Psychotherapy Relationships that Work: Evidence-based Responsiveness*, 2nd edn. Oxford: Oxford University Press.

Nouwen, H. (1992) *The Return of the Prodigal Son: A Story of Homecoming*. New York: Doubleday.

Oden, T. (1987) *Classical Pastoral Care, Vol. 3: Pastoral Counsel*. Grand Rapids, MI: Baker Books.

Ogden, T. (1986) *The Matrix of the Mind: Object Relations and the Psychoanalytic Dialogue*. Northvale, NJ: Jason Aronson.

Ogden, T. (1989) On the concept of an autistic-contiguous position, *International Journal of Psychoanalysis*, 70(1): 27–40.

Ogden, T. (1992) *Projective Identification and Psychotherapeutic Technique*. London: Karnac Books.

Ogden, T. (1994) The analytic third: working with intersubjective clinical facts, *International Journal of Psychoanalysis*, 75: 3–19.

Ogden, T. (2001) Reading Winnicott, *Psychoanalytic Quarterly*, 70: 299–323.

Ogden, T. (2013) The mother, the infant and the matrix, in J. Abram (ed.) *Donald Winnicott Today* (pp. 46–72). Hove: Routledge.

Orange, D. (2002) There is no outside: empathy and authenticity in psychoanalytic process, *Psychoanalytic Psychology*, 19(4): 686–700.

Orange, D. (2008) Whose shame is it anyway? Lifeworlds of humiliation and systems of restoration (or 'The Analyst's Shame'), *Contemporary Psychoanalysis*, 44(1): 83–100.

Orange, D. (2010) *Thinking for Clinicians: Philosophical Resources for Contemporary Psychoanalysis and the Humanistic Psychotherapies*. New York: Routledge.

Orange, D. (2011) *The Suffering Stranger: Hermeneutics for Everyday Clinical Practice*. New York: Routledge.

Orange, D. (2016) *Nourishing the Inner Life of Clinicians and Humanitarians*. Abingdon: Routledge.

Orange, D., Atwood, G. and Stolorow, R. (1997) *Working Intersubjectively: Contextualism in Psychoanalytic Practice*. Hillsdale, NJ: Analytic Press.

Page, S. (2010) *Diversity and Complexity*. Princeton, NJ: Princeton University Press.

Papadopoulos, R. (ed.) (2006) *The Handbook of Jungian Psychology: Theory, Practice and Applications*. London: Routledge.

Parsons. M. (2000) *The Dove that Returns, the Dove that Vanishes: Paradox and Creativity in Psychoanalysis*. London: Routledge.

Person, E. and Target, M. (eds.) (2013) *On Freud's 'Observations On Transference-Love'*. London: Karnac Books.

Pfister, O. [1928] (1993) The illusion of a future: a friendly disagreement with Prof. Sigmund Freud, *International Journal of Psychoanalysis*, 74 (3): 557–579.

Phillips, A. (1994) *On Flirtation*. London: Faber & Faber.

Pick, D. (2015) *Psychoanalysis: A Very Short Introduction*. Oxford: Oxford University Press.

Piontelli, A. (1992) *From Foetus to Child: An Observational and Psychoanalytic Study*. London: Routledge.

Price, J., Hilsenroth, M., Callahan, K., Petretic-Jackson, P. and Bonge, D. (2004) A pilot study of psychodynamic psychotherapy for adult survivors of childhood sexual abuse, *Clinical Psychology & Psychotherapy*, 11(6): 369–438.

Proctor, G. (2014) *Values and Ethics in Counselling and Psychotherapy*. London: SAGE.

Pollock, L. and Slavin, J. (1998) The struggle for recognition: disruption and reintegration in the experience of agency, *Psychoanalytic Dialogues*, 8(6): 857–873.

Pulver, S. (2001) On the astonishing clinical irrelevance of neuroscience, *Journal of the American Psychoanalytic Association*, 51(3): 1–18.

Pym, T. (1922) *Psychology and the Christian Life*. London: SCM Press.

Ramus, F. (2013) What's the point of neuropsychoanalysis?, *British Journal of Psychiatry*, 203(3): 170–171.

Raphael-Leff, J. (2015) *Dark Side of the Womb: Pregnancy, Parenting and Persecutory Anxieties*. London: Anna Freud Centre.

Rayner, E. (1991) *The Independent Mind in British Psychoanalysis*. Northvale, NJ: Jason Aronson.

Rees, L. (2017) *The Holocaust: A New History*. London: Viking.

Reeves, A. (2010) *Counselling Suicidal Clients*. London: SAGE.

Reeves, A. (2014) Research and individual therapy, in W. Dryden and A. Reeves (eds.) *The Handbook of Individual Therapy*, 6th edn. (pp. 577–601). London: SAGE.

Reisner, S. (1999) Freud and psychoanalysis: into the 21st century, *Journal of the American Psychoanalytic Association*, 47(4): 1037–1060.

Renn, P. (2012) *The Silent Past and the Invisible Present: Memory, Trauma, and Representation in Psychotherapy*. New York: Routledge.

Rizzolatti, G. and Craighero, L. (2004) The mirror-neuron system, *Annual Review of Neuroscience*, 27: 169–192.

Rodman, F.R. (ed.) (1987) *The Spontaneous Gesture: Selected Letters of D.W. Winnicott*. Cambridge, MA: Harvard University Press.

Rodman, F.R. (2003) *Winnicott: Life and Work*. Cambridge, MA: Perseus.

Rogers, C. (1951) *Client-centered Therapy: Its Current Practice, Implications, and Theory*. Boston, MA: Houghton Mifflin.

Rogers, C. (1961) *On Becoming a Person: A Therapist's View of Psychotherapy*. Boston, MA: Houghton Mifflin.

Rose, J. (2003) *On Not Being Able to Sleep: Psychoanalysis and the Modern World*. London: Chatto & Windus.

Ross, A. (1993) *An Evaluation of Clinical Theology 1958–1969*. Oxford: CTA.

Ross, A. (1997) *Evangelicals in Exile: Wrestling with Theology and the Unconscious*. London: DLT.

Ross, A. (2006) Psychodynamic counselling, religion and spirituality, in S. Wheeler (ed.) *Difference and Diversity in Counselling – Contemporary Psychodynamic Practice* (pp. 171–183). Basingstoke: Palgrave Macmillan.

Ross, A. (2010) Sacred psychoanalysis. PhD thesis, University of Birmingham.

Ross, A. (2014) A story of falling, *Therapy Today* (October).

Ross, A. (2016a) On learning from (being) the patient, *Psychodynamic Practice*, 22(3): 273–277.

Ross, A. (2016b) *Freud*, Pocket Giants Series. Stroud: The History Press.

Ross, A. (2016c) Spirituality and spiritual experiences in therapy, *Therapy Today* (May).

Ross, A. (2016d) Identifying the categories of spiritual experience encountered by therapists in their clinical work, *British Journal of Guidance and Counselling*, 44(3): 316–324.

Ross, A. (2016e) The power of a kiss, *Psychoanalytic Perspectives*, 13(3): 331–335.

Ross, A. (2018) Psychodynamic approaches, in A. Reeves (ed.) *An Introduction to Counselling and Psychotherapy: From Theory to Practice*, 2nd edn. (pp. 57–74). London: SAGE.

Ross, A. and Green, C. (2011) Inside the experience of anorexia nervosa: a narrative thematic analysis, *Counselling and Psychotherapy Research*, 11(2): 112–119.

Ross, A. and Loly, K. (2013) Grotstein's 'Black Hole' and working with borderline personality, *Psychodynamic Practice*, 19(4): 375–389.

Ross, J.M. (1999) Review of 'Ideas and Identities: The Life and Work of Erik Erikson' by R. Wallerstein and L. Goldberger, *Psychoanalytic Quarterly*, 68(4): 648–653.

Roth, A. and Fonagy, P. (2005) *What Works for Whom? A Critical Review of Psychotherapy Research*, 2nd edn. New York: Guilford Press.

Roth, A. and Pilling, S. (2007) *The Competences Required to Deliver Effective Cognitive and Behavioural Therapy for People with Depression and with Anxiety Disorders*. London: Department of Health.

Rowan, J. and Dryden, W. (eds.) (1988) *Innovative Therapy in Britain*. Buckingham: Open University Press.

Rucker, N. and Mermelstein, C. (1979) Unconscious communication in the mother–child dyad, *American Journal of Psychoanalysis*, 39(2):147–151.

Rustin, M. (2002) Looking in the right place: complexity theory, psychoanalysis and infant observation, *Infant Observation*, 5(1): 122–144.

Rustin, M. and Rustin, M. (2016) *Reading Klein*. Abingdon: Routledge.

Safran, J. (2012) *Psychoanalysis and Psychoanalytic Therapies*. Washington, DC: American Psychological Association.

Safran, J.D. and Muran, J.C. (2000) *Negotiating the Therapeutic Alliance: A Relational Treatment Guide*. New York: Guilford Press.

Safran, J.D., Muran, J.C. and Eubanks-Carter, C. (2011) Repairing alliance ruptures, *Psychotherapy*, 48: 80–87.

Samuels, A. (1985) *Jung and the Post-Jungians*. London: Routledge.

Sandell, R. (2012) Research on psychoanalysis and psychoanalytic-derived psychotherapies, in G. Gabbard, B. Litowitz and P. Williams (eds.) *Textbook of Psychoanalysis*, 2nd edn. (pp. 385–403). Washington, DC: American Psychiatric Publishing.

Sandell, R., Blomberg, J., Lazar, A., Carlsson, J., Broberg. J. and Schubert, J. (2000) Varieties of long-term outcome among patients in psychoanalysis and long-term psychotherapy: a review of findings in the Stockholm Outcome of Psychoanalysis and Psychotherapy Project (STOPP), *International Journal of Psychoanalysis*, 81: 921–942.

Sandler, A.-M. (2009) Commentary [see Friedman 2009], in P. Fonagy and M. Leuzinger-Bohleber (eds.) *Identity, Gender, and Sexuality: 150 Years After Freud* (pp. 98–102). London: Karnac Books.

Sayers, J. (1991) *Mothering Psychoanalysis*. London: Hamish Hamilton.

Sayers, J. (2003) *Divine Therapy: Love, Mysticism and Psychoanalysis*. Oxford: Oxford University Press.

Sayers, J. (2007) *Freud's Art – Psychoanalysis Retold*. London: Routledge.

Scalia, J. (ed.) (2002) *Vitality of Objects: Exploring the Work of Christopher Bollas*. London: Continuum.

Scarfone, D. (2013) A brief introduction to the work of Jean Laplanche, *International Journal of Psychoanalysis*, 94(3): 545–566.

Scarfone, D. (2015) *Laplanche: An Introduction*. New York: Unconscious in Translation.

Scarlett, J. (1991) Getting established: initiatives in psychotherapy training since World War Two, *British Journal of Psychotherapy*, 7: 260–267.

Schafer, R. (1977) The interpretation of transference and the conditions for loving, *Journal of the American Psychoanalytic Association*, 25: 335–362.

Schafer, R. (1995) In the wake of Heinz Hartmann, *International Journal of Psychoanalysis*, 76: 223–235.

Scharff, J. and Scharff, D. (eds.) (2005) *The Legacy of Fairbairn and Sutherland: Psychotherapeutic Applications*. London: Routledge.

Schimmel, P. (2014) *Sigmund Freud's Discovery of Psychoanalysis: Conquistador and Thinker*. London: Routledge.

Schore, A. (1994) *Affect Regulation and the Origin of the Self: The Neurobiology of Emotional Development*. Hillsdale, NJ: Erlbaum.

Schore, A. (2001) Minds in the making: attachment, the self-organizing brain, and developmentally-oriented psychoanalytic psychotherapy, *British Journal of Psychotherapy*, 17(3): 299–328.

Schore, A. (2003a) *Affect Dysregulation and Disorders of the Self*. New York: W.W. Norton.

Schore, A. (2003b) *Affect Regulation and the Repair of the Self*. New York: W.W. Norton.

Schore, A. (2011) The right brain implicit self lies at the core of psychoanalysis, *Psychoanalytic Dialogues*, 21: 75–100.

Schottenbauer, M., Glass, C., Arnkoff, D. and Gray, S. (2008) Contributions of psychodynamic approaches to treatment of PTSD and trauma: a review of the empirical treatment and psychopathology literature, *Psychiatry*, 71(1): 13–34.

Schredl, M., Bohusch, C., Kahl, J., Mader, A. and Somesan, A. (2000) The use of dreams in psychotherapy: a survey of psychotherapists in private practice, *Journal of Psychotherapy Practice and Research*, 9(2): 81–87.

Seligman, S. and Harrison, A. (2012) Infant research and adult psychotherapy, in G. Gabbard, B. Litowitz and P. Williams (eds.) *Textbook of Psychoanalysis*, 2nd edn. (pp. 239–252). Washington, DC: American Psychiatric Publishing.

Shamdasani, S. (2003) *Jung and the Making of Modern Psychology*. Cambridge: Cambridge University Press.

Shapiro, F. (2001) *Eye Movement Desensitization and Reprocessing: Basic Principles, Protocols, and Procedures*, 2nd edn. New York: Guilford Press.

Shapiro, Y. (2014) Psychodynamic formulation in the age of neuroscience: a dynamical systems model, *Psychoanalytic Dialogues*, 24(2): 175–192.

Shedler, J. (2010) The efficacy of psychodynamic psychotherapy, *American Psychologist*, 65(2): 98–109.

Shedler, J. (2017) Selling Bad Therapy to Trauma Victims. Available at: https://www.psychologytoday.com/blog/psychologically-minded/201711/selling-bad-therapy-trauma-victims [accessed 19 November 2017].

Shepherd, N. (1977) *The Living Mountain*. Aberdeen: Aberdeen University Press.

Shepherd, N. (2014) *In the Cairngorms*. Cambridge: Galileo Publishers.

Siegel, A. (1996) *Heinz Kohut and the Psychology of the Self*. London: Routledge.

Siegel, D. (1999) *The Developing Mind: Towards the Neurobiology of Interpersonal Experience*. New York: Guilford Press.

Siegel, D. (2012) *The Developing Mind: How Relationships and the Brain Interact to Shape Who We Are*, 2nd edn. New York: Guilford Press.

Sinason, V. (ed.) (2002) *Attachment, Trauma, and Multiplicity: Working Dissociative Identity Disorder*. Hove: Routledge.

Sinason, V. (ed.) (2012) *Trauma, Dissociations and Multiplicity: Working on Identity and Selves*. Hove: Routledge.

Slochower, J.A. (2014) *Holding and Psychoanalysis*, 2nd edn. London: Routledge.

Solms, M. (1997) *The Neuropsychology of Dreams: A Clinico-Anatomical Study*. Mahwah, NJ: Lawrence Erlbaum.

Solms, M. (2013) The unconscious in psychoanalysis and neuropsychology, in S. Akhtar and M.K. O'Neil (eds.) *On Freud's 'The Unconscious'* (pp. 101–118). London: Karnac Books.

Solms, M. and Leuzinger-Bohleber, M. (eds.) (2016) *The Unconscious: A Bridge Between Psychoanalysis and Cognitive Neuroscience*. London: Routledge.

Solms, M. and Turnball, O. (2011) What is neuropsychoanalysis?, *Neuropsychoanalysis*, 13(2): 1–13.

Solomon, H. (1994) The transcendent function and Hegel's dialectical vision, *Journal of Analytical Psychology*, 39 (1): 77–100.

Solomon, M. and Siegel, D. (eds.) (2003) *Healing Trauma: Attachment, Mind, Body, and Brain*. New York: W.W. Norton.

Spermon, D., Darlington, Y. and Gibney, P. (2010) Psychodynamic psychotherapy for complex trauma: targets, focus, applications, and outcomes, *Psychology Research and Behavior Management*, 3: 119–127.

Spezzano, C. (2012) Intersubjectivity, in G. Gabbard, B. Litowitz and P. Williams (eds.) *Textbook of Psychoanalysis*, 2nd edn. (pp. 103–116). Washington, DC: American Psychiatric Publishing.

Spillius, E. and O'Shaughnessy, E. (eds.) (2012) *Projective Identification: The Fate of a Concept*. Abingdon: Routledge.

Stefana, A. (2017) *History of Countertransference: From Freud to the British Object Relations School*. Abingdon: Routledge.

Stein, R. (2007) Moments in Laplanche's theory of sexuality, *Studies in Gender and Sexuality*, 8(2): 177–200.

Stern, D. (1985) *The Interpersonal World of the Infant*. New York: Basic Books.

Stern, D. (1995) *The Motherhood Constellation: A Unifying View of Parent–Infant Psychotherapy*. New York: Basic Books.

Stern, D. (1998) *The Interpersonal World of the Infant*, 2nd edn. New York: Basic Books.

Stern, D. (2004) *The Present Moment in Psychotherapy and Everyday Life*. New York: W.W. Norton.

Stern, D. and the Boston Change Process Study Group (2006) Some implications of infant observation for psychoanalysis, in A. Cooper (ed.) *Contemporary Psychoanalysis in America* (pp. 641–666). Washington, DC: American Psychiatric Publishing.

Stern, D., Sander, L.W., Nahum, J.P., Harrison, A.M., Lyons-Ruth, K., Morgan, A.C. et al. (1998) Non-interpretive mechanisms in psychoanalytic therapy: the 'something more' than interpretation, *International Journal of Psycho-Analysis*, 79: 903–921.

Stewart, H. (1996) *Michael Balint: Object Relations, Pure and Applied*. London: Routledge.

Strozier, C. (2001) *Heinz Kohut: The Making of a Psychoanalyst*. New York: Farrar, Straus & Giroux.

Summers, A. and Martindale, B. (2013) Using psychodynamic principles in formulation in everyday practice, *Advances in Psychiatric Treatment*, 19: 203–211.

Sutherland, J. (1989) *Fairbairn's Journey into the Interior*. London: Free Association Books.

Szekacs-Weisz, J. and Keve, T. (eds.) (2012a) *Ferenczi and His World: Rekindling the Spirit of the Budapest School*. London: Karnac Books.

Szekacs-Weisz, J. and Keve, T. (eds.) (2012b) *Ferenczi for Our Time: Theory and Practice*. London: Karnac Books.

Tang, Y., Hölzel, B. and Posner, M. (2015) The neuroscience of mindfulness meditation, *Nature Reviews Neuroscience*, 16: 213–225.

Tannahill, R. (1980) *Sex in History*. New York: Stein & Day.

Taylor, D. (2012) Psychoanalytic and psychodynamic therapies for depression: the evidence base, in R. Levy, J. Ablon and H. Kachele (eds.) *Psychodynamic Psychotherapy Research: Evidence-based Practice and Practice-based Evidence* (pp. 95–116). New York: Springer.

Thorne, B. (2007) Person-centred therapy, in W. Dryden (ed.) *Dryden's Handbook of Individual Therapy*, 5th edn (pp. 144–172). London: SAGE.

Timulak, L. (2009) *Research in Psychotherapy and Counselling*. London: SAGE.

Town, J.M., Diener, M.J., Abbass, A., Leichsenring, F., Driessen, E. and Rabung, S. (2012) A meta-analysis of psychodynamic psychotherapy outcomes: evaluating the effects of research-specific procedures, *Psychotherapy*, 49(3): 276–290.

Trevarthen, C. (1974) Conversations with a two-month-old, in J. Raphael-Leff (ed.) (2003) *Parent–Infant Psychodynamics: Wild Things, Mirrors and Ghosts* (pp. 25–34). London: Whurr Publishers.

Tronick, E. (1989) Emotions and emotional communication and infants, *American Psychologist*, 44(2): 112–119.

Tronick, E. (2007) *The Neurobiological and Social-emotional Development of Infants and Children*. New York: W.W. Norton.

Tronick, E. and Beeghly, M. (2011) Infants' meaning-making and the development of mental health problems, *American Psychologist*, 36(2): 107–119.

Ulnick, J. (2007) *Skin in Psychoanalysis*. London: Karnac Books.

Verhaeghe, P. (2009) *New Studies of Old Villains: A Radical Reconsideration of the Oedipus Complex*. New York: The Other Press.

Volkan, V. (2017) *Immigrants and Refugees: Trauma, Perennial Mourning, Prejudice, and Border Psychology*. London: Karnac Books.

Waddell, M. (2002) *Inside Lives: Psychoanalysis and the Growth of the Personality*, 2nd edn. London: Karnac Books.

Walker, M. (1992) *Surviving Secrets: The Experience of Abuse for the Child, the Adult and the Helper*. Buckingham: Open University Press.

Wallerstein, R. (1990) Psychoanalysis: the common ground, *International Journal of Psycho-Analysis*, 71: 3–20.

Wallwork, E. (2012) Ethics in psychoanalysis, in G. Gabbard, B. Litowitz and P. Williams (eds.) *Textbook of Psychoanalysis*, 2nd edn (pp. 349–366). Washington, DC: American Psychiatric Publishing.

Wampold, B. and Imel, Z. (2015) *The Great Psychotherapy Debate: The Evidence for What Makes Psychotherapy Work*, 2nd edn. New York: Routledge.

Wang, Q. and Peterson, C. (2014) Your earliest memory may be earlier than you think: prospective studies of children's dating of earliest childhood memories, *Developmental Psychology*, 50: 1680–1686.

Watkins, C.E., Jr. (2016) Psychoanalytic supervision in the new millennium: on pressing needs and impressing possibilities, *International Forum of Psychoanalysis*, 25(1): 50–67.

Watzke, B., Rüddel, H., Jürgensen, R., Koch, U., Kriston, L. and Grothgar, B. (2010) Effectiveness of systematic treatment selection for psychodynamic and cognitive-behavioural therapy: randomised controlled trial in routine mental healthcare, *British Journal of Psychiatry*, 197: 96–105.

Weatherill, R. (2017) *The Anti-Oedipus Complex: Lacan, Critical Theory and Postmodernism*. Abingdon: Routledge.

Webb, A. and Wheeler, S. (1998) How honest do counsellors dare to be in the supervisory relationship? An exploratory study, *British Journal of Guidance and Counselling*, 26(4): 509–524.

Weinberg, H. (2007) So what is this social unconscious anyway?, *Group Analysis*, 40(3): 307–322.

Weinstein, A. (2016) *Prenatal Development and Parents' Lived Experiences: How Early Events Shape Our Psychophysiology and Relationships*. New York: W.W. Norton.

Wheeler, S. (ed.) (2006) *Difference and Diversity in Counselling: Contemporary Psychodynamic Approaches*. Basingstoke: Palgrave Macmillan.

Wheeler, S. (2007) What shall we do with the wounded healer? The supervisor's dilemma, *Psychodynamic Practice*, 13(3): 245–256.

Wheeler, S. and Richards, K. (2007) The impact of clinical supervision on counsellors and therapists, their practice and their clients: a systematic review of the literature, *Counselling and Psychotherapy Research*, 7(1): 54–65.

Widlöcher, D. (2013) Winnicott and the acquisition of a freedom of thought, in J. Abram (ed.) *Donald Winnicott Today* (pp. 235–249). Hove: Routledge.

Wilkinson, M. (2006) *Coming into Mind. The Mind–Brain Relationship: A Jungian Clinical Perspective*. Hove: Routledge.

Wilkinson, M. (2010) *Changing Minds in Therapy: Emotion, Attachment, Trauma and Neurobiology*. New York: W.W. Norton.

Williams, J., Crane, C., Barnhofer, T., Brennan, K., Duggan, D., Fennell, M. et al. (2014) Mindfulness-based cognitive therapy for preventing relapse in recurrent depression: a randomized dismantling trial, *Journal of Consulting and Clinical Psychology*, 82(2): 275–286.

Williams, M. and Penman, D. (2011) *Mindfulness: A Practical Guide to Finding Peace in a Frantic World*. London: Piatkus.

Williams, M., Teasdale, J., Zindel, S. and Kabat–Zinn, J. (2007) *The Mindful Way Through Depression: Freeing Yourself from Chronic Unhappiness*. New York: Guilford Press.

Winnicott, D.W. (1949) Birth memories, birth trauma, and anxiety, in *Through Paediatrics to Psychoanalysis: Collected Papers*. London: Karnac Books.

Winnicott, D.W. (1955) Metapsychological and clinical aspects of regression within the psychoanalytical set-up, *International Journal of Psychoanalysis*, 36: 16–26.

Winnicott, D.W. (1956) On transference, *International Journal of Psychoanalysis*, 37: 386–388.

Winnicott, D.W. (1960) The theory of the parent–infant relationship, *International Journal of Psychoanalysis*, 41: 585–595.

Winnicott, D. W. [1947] (1964) Further thoughts on babies as persons, in *The Child, the Family, and the Outside World* (pp. 85–92). Harmondsworth: Penguin Books.

Winnicott, D.W. (1965) *The Maturational Processes and the Facilitating Environment: Studies in the Theory of Emotional Development*. London: Hogarth Press.

Winnicott, D. (2013) D.W.W. on D.W.W., in J. Abram (ed.) *Donald Winnicott Today* (pp. 29–45). Hove: Routledge.

Winnicott, D.W. (2016) *The Collected Works of D.W. Winnicott*, Vols. 1–12 (edited by L. Caldwell and H. Robinson). Oxford: Oxford University Press.

Woodward, J. (1998) *The Lone Twin: Understanding Twin Bereavement and Loss*. London: Free Association Books.

Yakeley, J. (2014) Psychodynamic psychotherapy: developing the evidence base, *Advances in Psychiatric Treatment*, 20: 269–279.

Index

Printed and bound by CPI Group (UK) Ltd, Croydon, CR0 4YY

12/06/2025

01900243-0013